Get Moving!

Wall Pilates for Seniors

To Improve

Fitness, Balance, Mobility & Strength

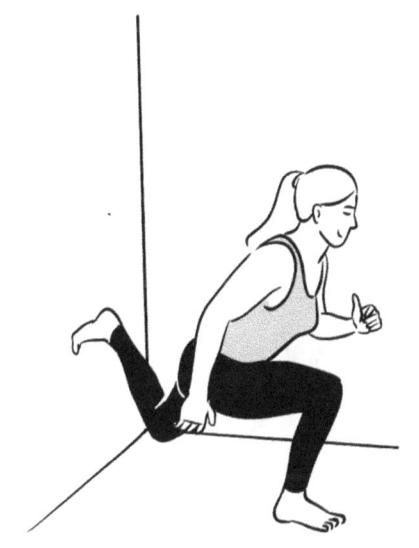

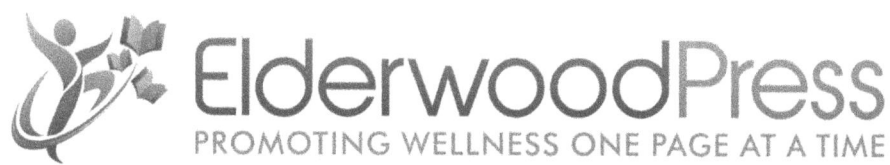

Copyright © 2025 by Elderwood Press, LLC

All rights reserved.

No portion of this book may be reproduced in any form without written permission from the publisher or author, except as permitted by U.S. copyright law.

Contents

A Personal Note	VII
1. How to Use This Book	1
2. Why Wall Pilates?	3
3. Dynamic Breathing Exercises	7
4. Warm-Up & Stretch Routines	9
5. Cardio, Metabolism & Strength	19
6. 28-Day Success Plan-Part 1 Days 1-14	23
7. 28-Day Success Plan-Part 2 Days 15-28	69
8. Easy Exercises for Strength, Fitness, and Weight Loss	119
9. Targeted Upper Body Exercises	127
10. Exercises for Balance & Coordination	133
11. Lower-Body Exercises	141
12. Exercises for Mobility and Independence	147
13. Our Gifts to You	155
Glossary	159
References	161

A Personal Note

I've always thought of myself as an active person; little league baseball and high school football growing up then jogging and bike riding as I got older. But out of nowhere at age 62, I was diagnosed with cancer. A devastating discovery at any age, but when you're over 60, it really makes you stop and think. I was fortunate to have some very capable doctors on my side who helped guide me and my family through the long and ominous treatment process.

While it's now under control, I didn't come out unscathed. The surgeries and chemotherapy took their toll. I started exercising again, but I was losing my battle with aches and pains, and my energy level was at an all-time low. Instead of making gains, I was pulling muscles, inflaming tendons and basically taking two steps back with each one forward.

Looking for something different, I tried Pilates, but it wasn't easy! It proved difficult for my lack of balance and flexibility. But, instead of quitting, I improvised. I used a chair for balance, a table for safety and the wall for stability. Then I realized that what I was doing was actually "**Wall Pilates**"; a low-impact exercise routine based around the wall and floor for support. I did some tweaking, assembled a few routines, and modified it all to be "senior friendly". That's how this book was born.

Wall Pilates now plays a significant role in my new health and fitness routine. I'm confident that if you embrace it like I have, you'll have a positive outcome, too. Please talk with your doctor before starting this program to make sure you have no underlying health issues that might not be compatible with exercise of this nature.

Welcome to your fitness journey. I'm glad you're here!

Sincerely,

Mike at Elderwood

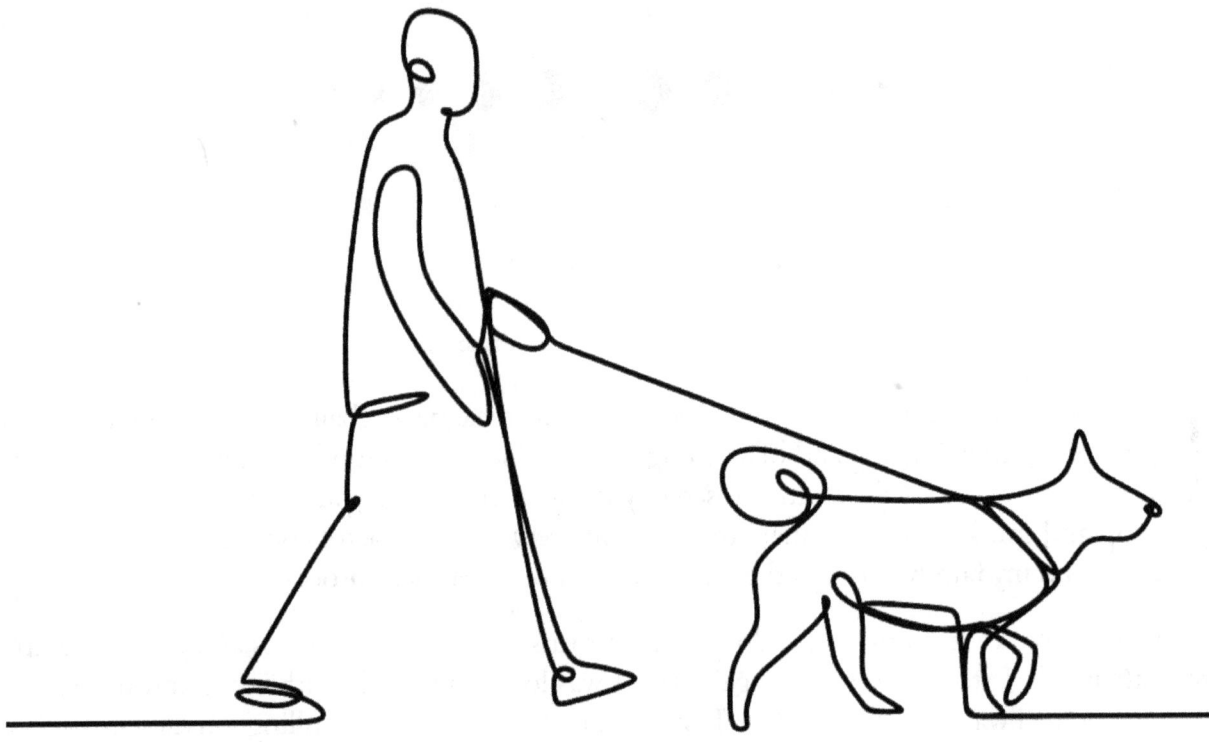

Chapter 1
How to Use This Book

Thank you for buying this book. "Get Moving! Wall Pilates for Seniors" is a comprehensive workout guide that makes your fitness journey fun and easy with routines designed for beginners and mature adults like us. It explains the "whys and hows" and gives specific exercises that can get you moving to increase your energy and strength, improve your balance, and help you lose those extra pounds. The centerpiece is a "28-Day Success Plan" with step-by-step routines for every day of the week and FREE VIDEO DEMONSTRATIONS to help you along the way. (See chapter 13 for access to the videos). It's the perfect workout solution for those looking to get moving again with fun and easy exercises especially for older adults and beginners.

Patience and Consistency: Your Keys to Success

When it comes to exercise, patience is of the essence. When you start out, your gains *will* be noticeable very quickly. But then, you might hit a plateau where it seems like you are getting nowhere. Remember you didn't get out of shape in a day, so real results won't come overnight. Keep pushing ahead. And be consistent. Exercise on a regular schedule. It's ok to take a day off to rest or do something else, but do something every day. If you don't feel like a regular routine, go for a fast walk, a swim, or a bike ride. Don't get comfortable doing "nothing". Once you stop, it's hard to get started again.

How to Use This Valuable Resource

Whether you're looking to reverse the results of a sedentary lifestyle, slow the effects of aging, or improve your fitness, your search ends here. This book takes traditional Pilates exercises and centers them around your wall. Some have you leaning, others lying down with your feet propped up, but they're all aimed at furthering your quest to get moving, lose weight, gain strength, and increase your balance and mobility. And it's not just a list of exercises and illustrations. We explain *why* you're doing the exercises and how they work together, not just *how* to do them.

This is a versatile workout program that adapts to your unique pace, providing a comfortable entry point for beginners and a sustainable progression for everyone. It starts with some background, so you can understand why you're doing what you're doing. After stretching and breathing routines, we walk you through the 28-Day Success Plan: a two-part, step-by-step daily guide with specific exercises to follow for 28 days. In later chapters, we group exercises into the body areas they primarily work (upper body, lower body, core, etc.) or with specific objectives in mind (cardio health, greater strength, improving balance, for instance). Use these *after* the 28-Day Plan to work toward your particular goals.

Bonus: Free Illustration Chart and Video Demonstrations

To ensure your absolute success, see Chapter 13 for instructions on how to get your ***free video demonstrations*** and the chart of illustrations used in this book. They show you how to perform each exercise and complement the descriptions outlined here. Take a few minutes to watch the videos to familiarize yourself with the moves, or dive right in and refer back to the videos when you need extra help. Either way, they're our free gifts to you to keep you moving forward.

Guided Audiobook Available Soon!

For a voice-guided workout, the audiobook version will be available soon on Audible. Visit our website for more information: www.ElderwoodPress.com.

Finally, if you want to skip all the background chatter and get right to it, feel free to skip to the warm-up and stretching exercises in Chapter 4. Welcome to the new you.

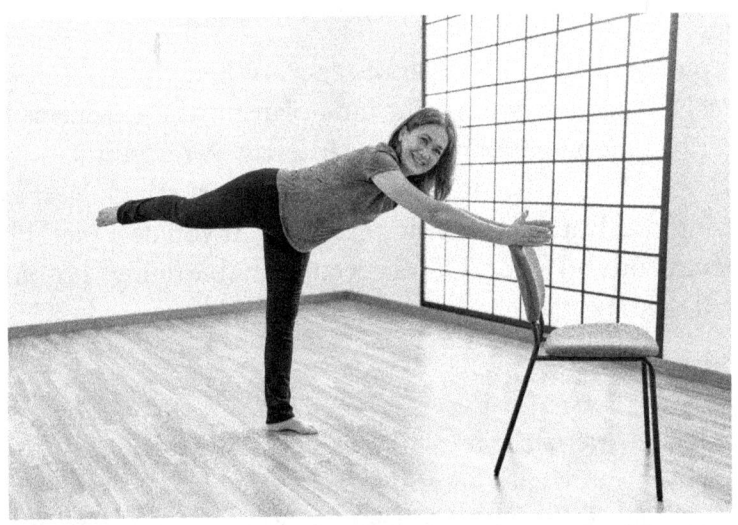

Chapter 2
Why Wall Pilates?

Fifty years ago, people were more active. Jobs were strenuous and kept us moving all day long. Over the last half-century, there has been a dramatic shift from physically demanding occupations to more sedentary service jobs. In the early 1960s, almost half of private industry jobs required at least moderately intensive physical activity. Today, less than 20% of us are involved in this level of moving around. Many of us are at a desk all day and as a result, the average person gets up to one-fifth less exercise from what we do all day than our counterparts of the past. To counteract this loss, we have to consciously make time for exercise.

Exercise and Growing Older

You might think that as the years go by, exercise becomes more of a spectator sport than an active one. I believe that age is just a number, and that exercise doesn't check your ID at the door. It's the universal secret to feeling fantastic at any age. You're not too old to groove, move, and unleash your inner fitness warrior! It's your ticket to a healthier, happier you. Regular exercise can help improve your mood, produce sleep better, and give you an energy boost that just might have you wondering if you've found the fountain of youth.

But, let's be honest; starting any type of new exercise program can feel a little intimidating, even if you're excited to begin and looking forward to the benefits. If, like me, you've somehow found yourself in your "mature adulthood" (how did that happen so fast?), then you might even be thinking about old dogs and impossible new tricks. Well, have no fear because that's the great thing about Wall Pilates. It's relatively easy to learn and fun to do. It doesn't take fancy equipment, or a pricy gym membership. To practice Wall Pilates, all you need is a wall and a willingness to stretch your comfort zone with a new spin on some established exercises. Take a step towards greater flexibility, better balance, and increased strength with Wall Pilates.

It Was all Greek to Me

Pilates sounds like a fancy made-up name, but the exercise was actually named after the guy who started it all in the early 1900's, Joseph Pilates. He was into fitness before it was cool and was considered an early adopter of work outs to promote body and mind health. Today, you can find Pilates classes and studios worldwide. *Wall Pilates* is an adaptation of the traditional exercise where the wall is used for safety and to ease the strain on those who find traditional Pilates too difficult or stenuous.

The Pilates Principles

Wall Pilates shares the six basic principles with traditional Pilates: Centering, Concentration, Control, Precision, Breath, and Flow.

Centering means to draw your energy from the physical center of your body, which we define as the core and pelvic floor muscles.

Concentration is to be fully present and focused in each movement of each exercise.

Control and Precision go hand-in-hand. To make clean, precise movements, you must control your muscles and movements. Difficult at first, this gets easier as your body adapts to your new flexibility and your comfort level increases. Sloppy moves and overly quick movements are counter-productive and not encouraged.

Breath is easily dismissed by beginners, but it's an important part of the process. Deliberate breathing ensures a constant flow of oxygen to purge the body's impurities, and delivers energy to the working muscles. It also helps you concentrate and be fully present during your exercises.

The last principle, **Flow,** is all about the importance of sequencing. Movements and exercises should flow seamlessly between each other.

The Basic Benefits of Wall Pilates

Traditional Pilates workouts normally take place in a gym on menacing machines with names like "The Reformer" and "Trapeze Table." It tends to be somewhat intimidating for those of us with less experience who may want to start slower. But Wall Pilates simplifies our workouts by using the wall for balance, added resistance, and, in some cases, safety, resulting in straightforward yet surprisingly effective exercise routines. Back, shoulders, neck, legs, core, and more; these routines work the entire body. And done right, they can even provide cardio benefits! It *demands* that we single-task to do it effectively, producing results in our bodies ***and*** our minds.

The Transformative Benefits

Here are some specific gains you might expect when you earnestly apply yourself to a Wall Pilates Program:

Strength and fitness. We've designed these sequences to get your heart beating, blood flowing and muscles working. This can contribute to greater strength and better overall fitness.

Enhanced balance. Since the CDC reports that falls are a leading cause of injury for older adults, you can't go wrong with wanting to decrease your chances of taking a tumble.

Improved posture. When your body is better aligned, you'll experience less aching, stiffness, and pressure on your joints.

A stronger core. When you're stronger through the core, you can better support yourself in your daily activities.

Weight management. Increased activity and the low-impact training in Wall Pilates helps you burn calories and build lean muscle, which can help boost your metabolism.

Increased energy levels. Wall Pilates helps foster improved respiratory function and better circulation meaning more oxygen getting where it needs to be, quicker.

Mindful eating habits. More informed food choices can help increase your metabolism and manage weight and nutrition.

Our focus on control and precision translates into fewer exercises that have greater benefits overall. The American Geriatrics Society says that incorporating different types of exercise into our routines (aerobic, strength training, balance, and flexibility) can maximize our health benefits as we age. Wall Pilates is perfect for this. And, because it uses the wall as a stabilizing partner, it's wonderful if you're concerned with your balance. Having the wall as both a support system and an immovable source of tactile feedback for correcting posture and alignment helps make Wall Pilates safe and easy to do.

If all of this sounds appealing, then Wall Pilates could be your key to better physical and mental health. Before you get started, be sure to download the reference chart and watch the videos for further clarification on how to perform any of the exercises. Instructions on how to access them can be found in Chapter 13. Now, on to the next chapter, where we'll explore the power of controlled breathing.

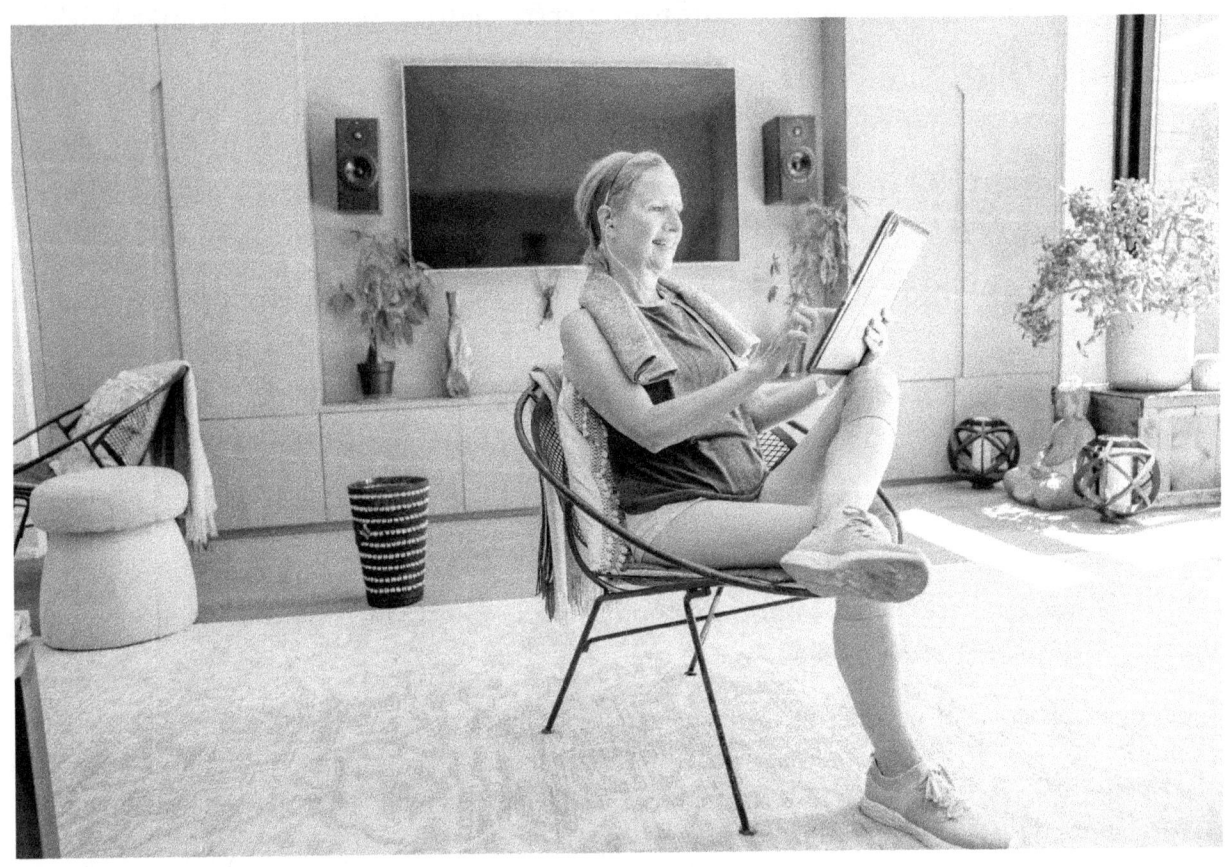

Chapter 3
Dynamic Breathing Exercises

• • • ● • ● • ● • • •

Think about this: the average person takes about 20 thousand breaths each day. That's enough air to blow up 4,000 party balloons. And we do it all day, every day without thinking. Imagine if we were conscious of our breathing. That would be kind of irritating for 24 hours a day, but can be very useful during exercise. During exercise, how we breathe is just as important as how we move, which makes breathing a critical component of exercise.

Let's call this "mindful breathing". Mindful breathing can greatly affect both physical and mental health by oxygenating the blood, reducing stress, and improving focus during exercise and beyond. It's fundamental to achieving the full benefits of workouts by refreshing our lungs and helping us focus on what we're doing at that moment.

Breathing and Exercise

With Wall Pilates, it's important to breathe deeply and rhythmically. Inhale through the nose, allowing your ribcage to expand. As you exhale through your mouth, use your core muscles to pull your navel in towards your spine. This helps keep your core stable while you take full, deep breaths. Focusing on your breath, you help make each movement more intentional and effective, amplifying the exercise benefits.

Mindful breathing on its own can also bring many of the same positive results as it does while exercising. Regular breathing practice can also help your focus and increase your energy. To that end, we've come up with a few specific breathing exercises you can try. Pick your favorites, sprinkle them throughout the day, and see how they make you feel. I've found them a great way to gently ease me into my workouts, helping me focus on the routines ahead. So, take a deep breath, and here we go.

Belly Breathing for Breath Control. To start, sit comfortably with your back straight. Place one hand on your chest and the other on your belly. Breathe in deeply through the nose, allowing your belly to expand while keeping your chest still. Hold momentarily and then exhale slowly through your mouth, drawing your belly inward. Breathe in; breathe out. Pay specific attention to your belly's rise and fall. Continue for about two minutes.

Ocean Sounding Breath for Concentration. Slowly inhale through your nose and then exhale through your mouth while slightly constricting the back of the throat, producing a soft sound like you're fogging a pane of glass or a mirror. Repeat slowly 10 times.

Box Breathing for Stress Relief & Discipline. Sit upright comfortably. Inhale through the nose slowly while counting to four in your head. Hold that breath for a count of four. Exhale through the mouth for a count of four. Hold that breath out for another count of four. Complete 5-10 cycles.

Nostril Yoga Breathing for Calm & Stress Relief. Begin by closing your right nostril with your right thumb and inhaling through your left nostril. Next, close your left nostril with your ring finger, releasing your right nostril. Exhale through the right nostril. Inhale through the right nostril, close it with your right thumb, then exhale through the left nostril. This is one cycle; complete four.

Laughter Breath for Stress Relief. Take a few deep breaths through the nose and out through the mouth. Then, start a "fake" laugh, forcefully exhaling as the laughter comes out. Think of a funny moment or situation and allow this fake laugh to turn into real, hearty laughter. Let the laughter roll for a bit, then return to deep breathing. Continue for 1-2 minutes.

Cooling Breath for Physical Cooling. This technique can have a calming effect on the nervous system. Sit upright, ensuring your posture is open but relaxed. Stick your tongue out and roll it like a tube. Inhale through this tubular tongue. Close your mouth and exhale normally through the nose. Repeat ten cycles.

Hissing Breath for Concentration. The "hissing" is a focal point, making concentrating on the breath and clearing the mind easier. To start, inhale deeply through the nose then exhale slowly through clenched teeth, creating a hissing sound as the air escapes. Repeat five times.

Ujjaya Breath for Physical Warming (Pronounced: "ooo-jaw-ee"). Sit comfortably with your back straight but not rigid. Inhale deeply through the nose. Keep your mouth and lips closed and exhale through your nose, creating a sound similar to whispering. Repeat five to ten times.

Humming Breath for Calm & Stress Relief. Start by finding a comfortable but upright position in your chair. Close your eyes and take a slow, deep breath through the nose. Exhale slowly through your mouth while producing a humming sound. Repeat ten times.

Incorporating these stand-alone breathing techniques into your day can significantly enhance your overall energy and concentration. As you continue to explore and refine these techniques, you may discover a renewed sense of vitality and well-being that extends far beyond your workout sessions.

CHAPTER 4
Warm-Up & Stretch Routines

• • • • ● • ● • • • •

You've probably had those days when you didn't feel like getting out of bed. But, once you put those feet on the floor and take your first steps, it gets a lot easier. Trying to exercise without mentally preparing and warming up first is like being in a warm bed on a cold morning. You have to convince yourself it's worth it. With exercise, if your mind isn't into it, your body isn't far behind.

How Warm-Ups and Stretching Help

Blood flow. When you exercise, your body wants to get more blood and oxygen to the muscles, but your body isn't ready immediately. That's where warm-ups come in. We're telling the body to gradually increase the resources responsible for the rise in blood flow. As we slowly raise the body's workload, blood vessels tend to dilate, allowing more blood to flow through. So, even simple muscle movements (like stretching and warm-ups) can positively impact your subsequent workout results *before you even start your routine.*

Flexibility and range of motion. Warm-ups help loosen your joints by increasing their "lubricating oil" (Synovial Fluid) and stretch muscles by gradually raising the body's core temperature, making them more pliable and responsive. This helps us to move more easily and with better technique, reducing the chance of injury. By activating the central nervous system, warm-ups can also **improve coordination and balance**, decrease **reaction time, and increase mental focus.** The dynamic movements and increased blood flow during a warm-up prepare you and your body for the upcoming workout.

Let's try a few warm-up stretches and start getting familiar with the exercises we'll be doing in this book. These all-body moves are perfect for an early morning routine to get your day going. We've outlined three separate routines here. Make sure you alternate between them to do a different routine each time.

Warm-Up Set 1

Tricep/Scapula Stretch
Works: Shoulders, Chest, Spine, Upper Back
Benefits: Warm-up & Flexibility

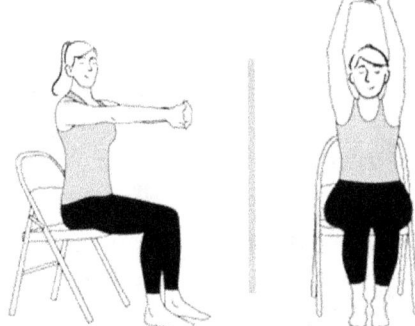

Instructions
Stand facing away from the wall and raise your left arm overhead. Bend your elbow so your arm is behind your head and your hand is on your upper back. Use your right arm to pull the elbow closer to your head and push down slightly. Allow your muscles to gently release as you hold the stretch for 30 seconds.
Repeat with the opposite arm.

The Scoop
Works: Shoulders, Chest, Spine, Upper Back
Benefits: Posture, Flexibility, Breathing

Instructions
Interlock your fingers and inhale as you bring them towards your chin. Exhale slowly as you straighten your elbows and turn your interlocked palms outward until your arms are fully extended. Keep the motion going as you raise your hands above your head with your palms towards the ceiling. Release your hands, turn your palms out, and bring them slowly to your sides. Repeat five times.

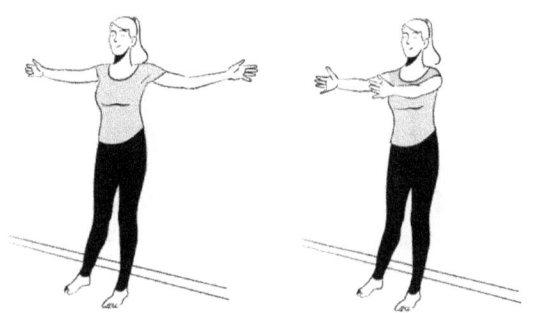

Bird Flap
Works: Scapula, Chest, Shoulders
Benefits: Flexibility, Balance

Stand with your back to the wall, with your feet two feet away. Spread your arms like an airplane, with the backs of your arms touching the all and your palms facing out. Keeping your elbows locked, bring your arms straight out in front of you so that your thumbs are up and your palms are facing each other and nearly touching. Hold briefly and return. That's one. Repeat at a medium speed 15 times for two sets.

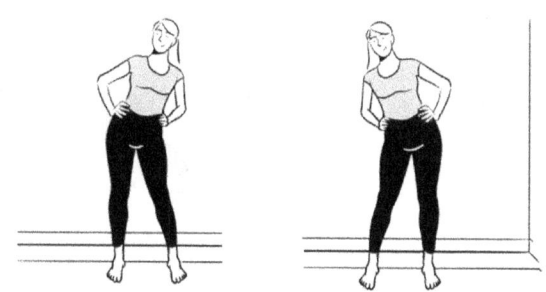

Large Hip Circles
Works: Hips, Upper Legs
Benefits: Flexibility, Mobility Balance, Strength

Stand facing the wall, with your feet shoulder-width apart about two feet from the wall. Put your hands on the hips and pull your stomach in to engage your core muscles. Bend to the side slightly and rotate your hips clockwise 10 times at a medium speed. Repeat in the other direction. Increase the size of the circles as you become more flexible and comfortable with the exercise.

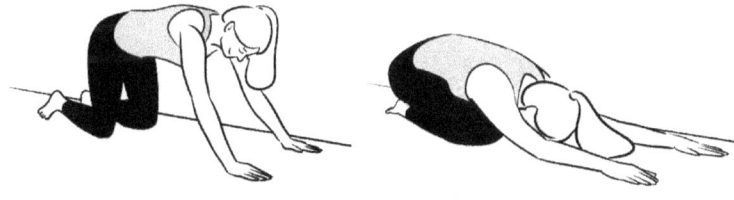

Child's Pose
Works: Shoulders, Legs, Back
Benefits: Flexibility, Mobility Independence, Strength

Start on hands and knees wit your arms stretched out slightly in front. Bend back, bending your knees and folding your upper body so you are almost sitting on your legs. Stretch out your arms with your palms on the floor. Hold for 20 seconds.

Wall Oblique Twist

Works: Upper Lats, Abdominals
Benefits: Flexibility, Mobility
Independence, Strength

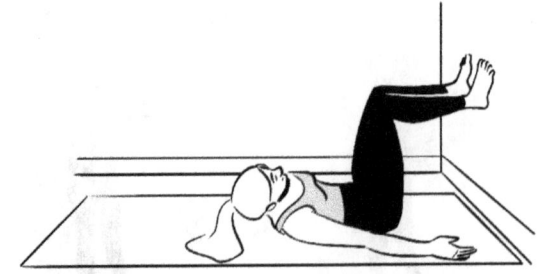

Lie on your back with your hands at your sides, your feet on the wall and your knees bent to form a 90-degre angle. Keeping your arms near the floor, lift your head and neck slightly, bend them to the right as you reach your right hand towards the wall without arching your back. Hold for three seconds and return to neutral position. Repeat on the left side.

Butterfly

Works: Hamstring, Quadricepts, Groin
Benefits: Flexibility, Mobility
Balance, Warm-Up

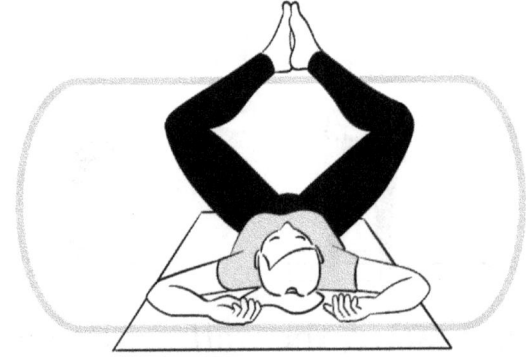

Sit with your right side next to the wall. Swing your legs up against the wall while turning to lie on your back and placing your hips against the wall. Bend your elbows and let your arms rest above your head on the mat. Keeping your feet on the wall, bend your knees in toward your chest while lowering your heels as low as you can and putting the soles of your feet together. Stay in this position for two to three minutes.

End of Warm-Up Set #1. Turn the page for set 2.

Warm-Up Set 2

Cactus Arms

Works: Back, Chest, Shoulders
Benefits: Flexibility, Warm-Up

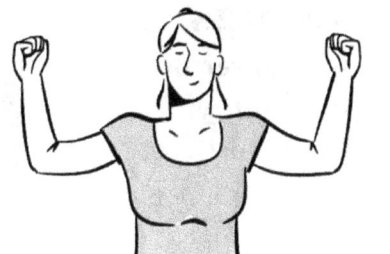
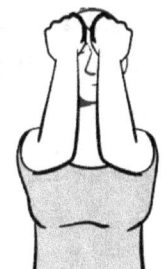

Start with your back and body against the wall. Extend your arms straight out from your sides like an airplane and bend up at the elbow like a cactus. The back of your hands and forearms should be touching the wall. With arms still bent, move them forward so that your palms and forearms come together in front of you. Hold for three second and return to start. Repeat 15 times.

Single Arm Pec Stretch

Works: Back, Chest, Shoulders
Benefits: Flexibility, Warm-Up

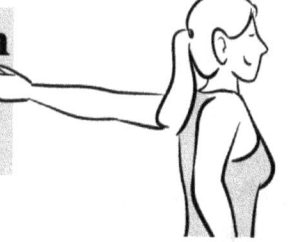
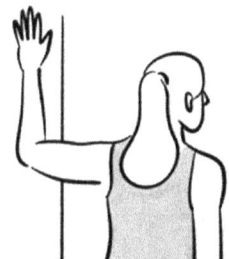

This exercise can be done with your arm extended or bent at the elbow. For arm extended, stand facing the wall an arm's length away. Lift your left arm to shoulder height, place your palm on the wall and twist your body gently to the right. Hold for ten seconds. Focus on feeling a stretch in the chest and shoulders. Repeat the stretch on the opposite side. For bent arm, bend your arm at the elbow.

Standing Wall Stretch

Works: Back, Chest, Shoulders
Benefits: Flexibility, Warm-Up

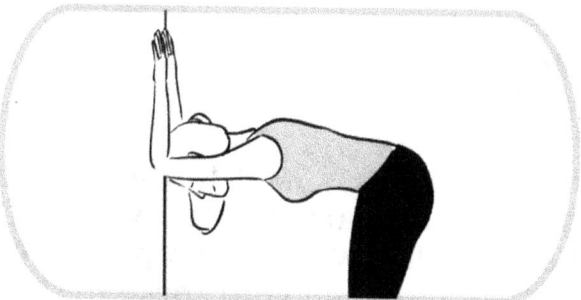

Stand about half an arm's length away and facing the wall. Keeping your legs straight, bend at the hips and put your elbows and forearms on the wall as you breathe out. Hold for 5-10 seconds.

Lateral Leg Swings
Works: Hips, Glutes, Lower Body
Benefits: Flexibility, Mobility, Balance & Strength

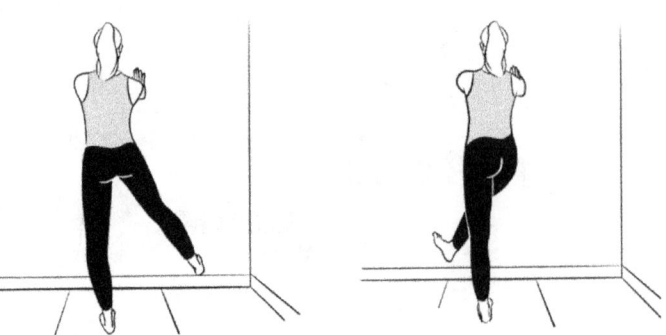

Stand straight with your palms on the wall. Exhale and swing your right leg laterally in front of your left leg towards your left side. Inhale as you return. Do this ten times then repeat with the left leg.

Single Leg Circles
Works: Legs, Hips, Core
Benefits: Flexibility, Mobility

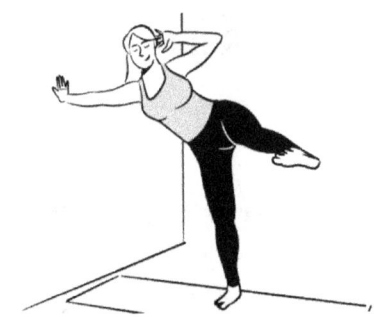

Put your left hand on the wall about 1 1/2 arm's lengths away and your right hand on the back of your head with your elbow bent. Bend slightly at the hips and keeping your left leg straight, make wide circles with your right leg. Repeat five times in each direction then switch legs.

Side Bend/Side Stretch
Works: Obliques, Lats
Benefits: Flexibility & Mobility

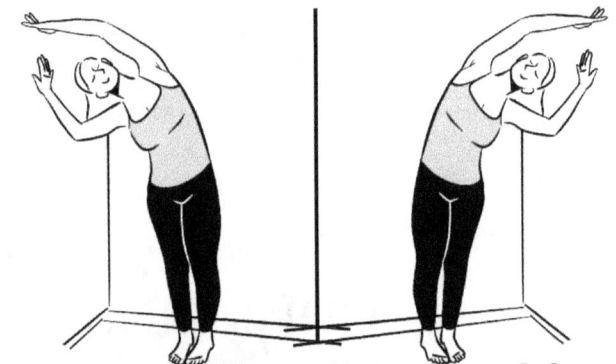

Stand sideways next to the wall, with your right side closest and feet hip-width apart. Extend your left arm overhead, placing your right hand on the wall for support. Gently slide your right hand down the wall as you bend your torso to the right, feeling a stretch along the left side of your body. Hold for 30 seconds then switch sides.

WARM-UP & STRETCH ROUTINES   15

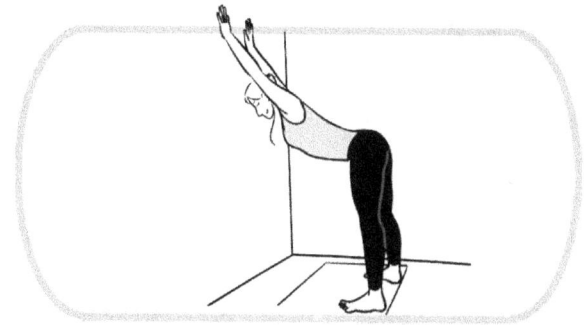

Arms Overhead

Works: Chest, Shulders, Upper Back
Benefits: Flexibility & Strength

Stand facing the wall, an arm's length away. Raise your arms over your head and place your palms flat against the wall. Keeping your arms straight, lean forward and press your chest towards the wall until you feel a stretch in your upper chest. Hold the stretch for 20 to 30 seconds, then relax and repeat. For more difficulty, put your palms together as you raise your arms.

Sit Stretch

Works: Back, Shoulders, Waist, Legs
Benefits: Flexibility, Mobility
Strength

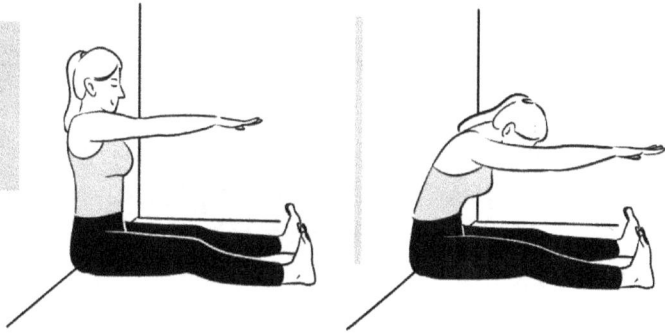

Sit on the floor with your back touching the wall and your arms straight out in front of you. Slowly bend forward, bending at the waist with your head pointed so you are looking at the floor. Go as far as you feel comfortable and hold for thirty seconds. Release and repeat, this time going farther than the first and again holding for thirty seconds.

End of Warm-up set #2. Keep going for set 3.

Warm-Up Set 3

Wall Angels
Works: Back, Neck, Shoulders
Benefits: Flexibility, Mobility, Strength

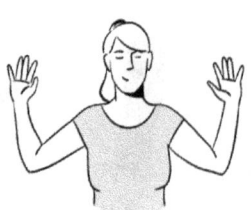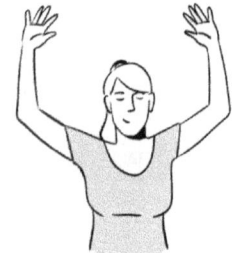

Stand with your back to the wall and feet about six inches away. Bend your arms 90 degrees while keeping them as flat against the wall as possible and slowly raise them arms up as far as possible. Use your abs to press your back against the wall. Hold for three seconds at the top then bring back down. Repeat five times.

Arm Rolls
Works: Shoulders, Back
Benefits: Flexibility, Cardio

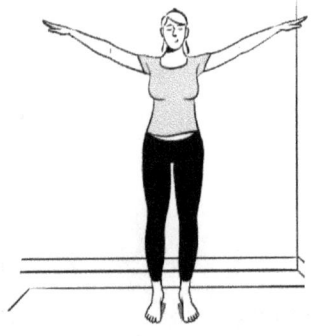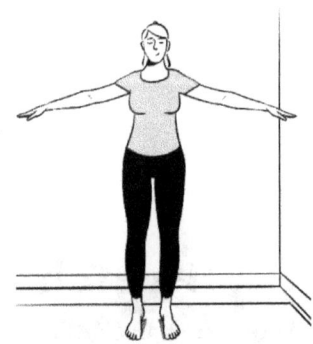

Stand about three feet from the wall, legs shoulder length apart and your arms out like an airplane. Keeping your elbows locked, make large, forward circles with your arms at medium speed. Do this five times then switch directions for five more repetitions. Repeat in each direction five times.

Large Front Arm Circles
Works: Shoulders, Obliques, Lats
Benefits: Flexibility & Mobility

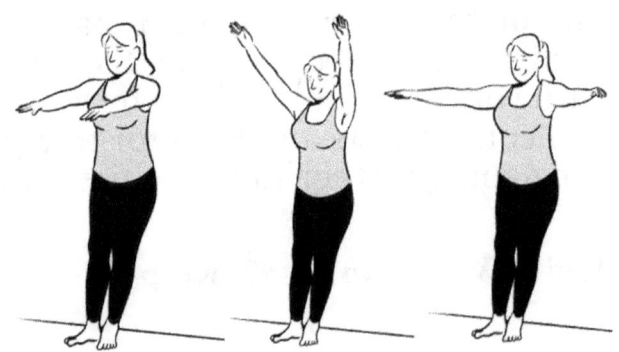

With your back against the wall, bend your knees slightly, raise your arms in front with your elbows locked. Raise them above your head then out to your sides like an airplane and then down. That's one circle. Do ten slow circles, reverse motion then do ten more.

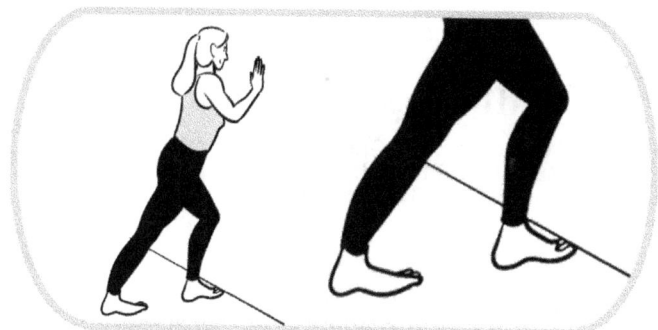

Calf Stretch
Works: Calves
Benefits: Warm-up, Stretching

Stand facing the wall about one and a half arm lengths away, feet shoulder length apart. Lean forward to the wall, bend your left knee as you slide the right foot back, keeping it flat on the floor until you feel the stretch in your calf. Hold for 10 seconds and release. Return to start and repeat with the opposite leg and calf.

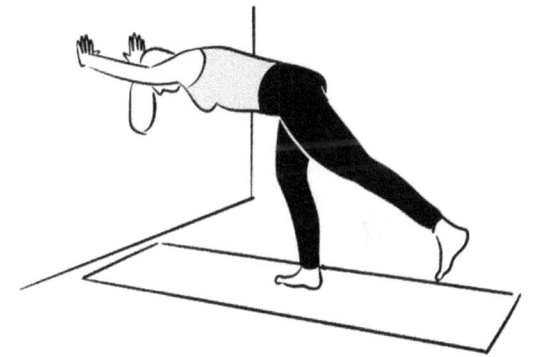

Rear Leg Lifts
Works: Hamstring, Hips, Spine
Benefits: Flexibility, Mobility, Balance, Strength

Face the wall an arm's length away. Bend at the waist, keep your body straight and put your palms on the wall, bending until your body forms an "L". Swing your right leg out behind and up as far as you comfortably can. Hold for a second then bring it back to the start. That's one. Repeat 10 times then switch to the left leg for 10 more.

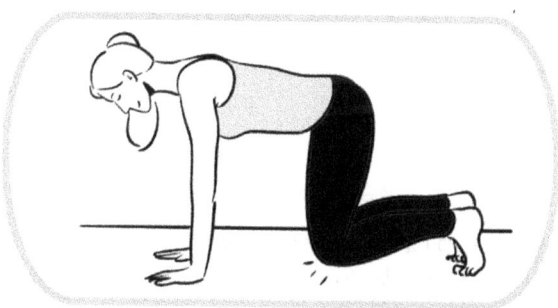

Knee Hover
Works: Abs, Core
Benefits: Balance & Strength

Kneel on the floor sideways from the wall with your back straight and your toes on the floor. Pick both knees up off the floor about one inch and hold for 30 seconds. Relax briefly then repeat five times.

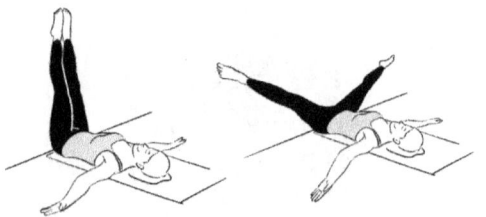

Wall Scissors
Works: Abs, Glutes, Inner Thighs
Benefits: Flexibility, Mobility, Balance & Strength

Lay on your side with your legs bent and against the wall. Roll over onto your back so that your legs and buttocks are up against the wall. Stretch your arms out from your side like an airplane. Open your legs widely to stretch the inner thigh and hold for two seconds. Bring back to neutral. Repeat 10 times.

Tabletop Reach
Works: Shoulders, Hips, Glutes
Benefits: Flexibility, Mobility Strength

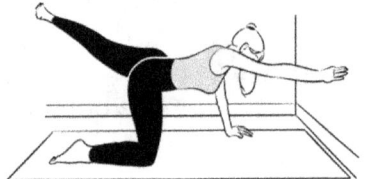 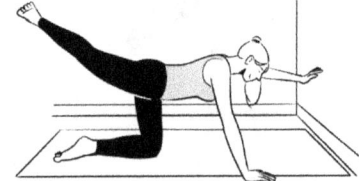

Start on your hands and knees facing the wall about an arm's length away. Extend your left leg straight back with toes pointed straight as you simultaneously reach out to the wall with your right hand. Return to the neutral position and then extend your right leg out and touch the wall with your left hand. Do this in a rapid, smooth succession five to ten times alternating sides each time.

These warm-up exercises are good for a morning wake-up call or any time you need a little energy during the day. In the next chapter, we'll take a quick look at the interplay between cardio, metabolism, and strength and how Wall Pilates can optimize each one, helping you meet your fitness goals. Then, we'll venture into the 28-Day Success Plan. Later, we'll show you targeted exercises to meet your specific goals. See you in Chapter 5.

Chapter 5
Cardio, Metabolism & Strength

Cardiovascular Conditioning (or heart health) is important if we want to be healthy, feel good, and continue to be independent. As we get older, our cardiovascular systems undergo changes that can increase the risk of heart-related issues. Things like:

-**Stiffening of blood vessels** (arteriosclerosis), which reduces blood flow. My mother used to call this "hardening of the arteries";

-**Thickening of heart muscle walls**, which can decrease pumping efficiency;

-**Increased risk of irregular heartbeats** like atrial fibrillation, which can cause a stroke;

-**A higher likelihood** of developing high blood pressure.

All this sounds scary, but it doesn't have to be depressing. Regular exercise can help us avoid these issues by potentially strengthening the heart muscle and improving blood circulation, lowering blood pressure and cholesterol levels, and improving our endurance and overall fitness levels. It has the added benefit of helping us manage our weight, which can also reduce the risk of heart disease. If you take medicine for a health issue, ***do not stop taking the medicine***. Please talk to your doctor before starting any exercise program (including this one) or before changing your medicine routine.

The Metabolism Shift

Our metabolism works together in a loop with our cardiovascular or "cardio" system (the heart and everything attached to it). It provides the energy needed for the heart system to work, while the heart system gives the metabolism what *it* needs to work properly. This interplay is fundamental to maintaining overall health and adapting to changing body conditions.

The metabolism is like the body's engine, where a series of chemical reactions turn the food we eat into energy and building blocks for growth while also getting rid of waste. As we get older, it tends to slow down, making weight management a bit trickier than it used to be.

At the same time, our muscles start to shrink-whether we like it or not! Scientists call this process "Sarcopenia"-and the older we get, the faster it goes. Without exercise, we can lose up to a third of our muscles by the time we're 70. And weaker muscle strength can lead to weaker bones, Osteoporosis, falls and injuries. Starting or continuing exercise as we age can help slow Sarcopenia and keep our bone density where it needs to be.

Types of exercises and how they help

All movement is not created equal. It's essential that we do the right exercises to work different areas for a balanced body.

- **Aerobic Exercise** is where the heartbeat is elevated for a longer period of time. It improves cardiovascular endurance and lung function by strengthening the cardiovascular system that carries blood and oxygen throughout our bodies. It also helps manage weight through calorie burn and reduces the risk of heart disease. **Remember-ALWAYS consult your doctor** before starting an exercise program that focuses on an elevated heart rate.

- **Strength Training Exercises** build and maintain muscle, increase bone density to reduce the risk of osteoporosis and improve balance and coordination, reducing our fall risk.

- **Flexibility Exercises** help increase joint mobility and range of motion, improve posture and reduce stress to promote relaxation.

The good news is that the routines in this book are designed to work all of these areas in a fun and productive way! This is our "holistic approach" and can lead to better overall physical function, independence, and quality of life. With Wall Pilates, it's important to remember that all exercises work together to bring overall strength to the body. That means that any "strength" exercises you perform also contribute to helping your balance, flexibility, and overall fitness. To understand this, let's take a quick look at how metabolism, strength, and weight loss are all intertwined.

Metabolism is how the body converts food into energy. Our bodies need a minimum amount of energy just to perform basic functions, even when we're resting. Muscles play a significant role in this. The higher our muscle mass, the more calories our bodies need to function because muscle tissue requires more energy to maintain itself than fat tissue. This means that the more muscle we have, the more calories we'll burn while we're just hanging out. So, our main goal should be building and maintaining our muscles.

When we exercise, the heart gets a workout, but more importantly, the blood vessels, veins, and arteries that supply the heart also benefit. Regular exercise builds these transport systems to make sure our hearts and bodies get what they need to do the work we're asking them to do without too much strain.

How Much is Enough?

If you want to burn more calories even when resting, you'll want to build muscle and work on your cardio. Here are some general recommendations:

- **Aerobic Exercise:** At least 150 minutes per week of moderate-intensity aerobic activity (like fast walking, swimming, or bicycling), or 75 minutes per week of high-intensity aerobic activity (like running, hiking, or sports), or a combination of these two. Base the intensity, duration, and recovery on your current fitness level, factoring in any cardiovascular conditions you might have. Talk to your doctor before starting any exercise routine.

- **Strength Training:** Practice exercises targeting all the major muscle groups at least twice a week. Try and do 8-12 repetitions of each exercise, using a resistance or stretch that challenges you. Increase the resistance as your body responds, and it gets easier.

These general guidelines can vary based on your health, fitness level, and personal goals. Always talk with your doctor before beginning any new exercise program or increasing your intensity. Now that we've explored the theory behind the movements and tried some breathing and stretching, it's time to start the "28-Day Success Plan".

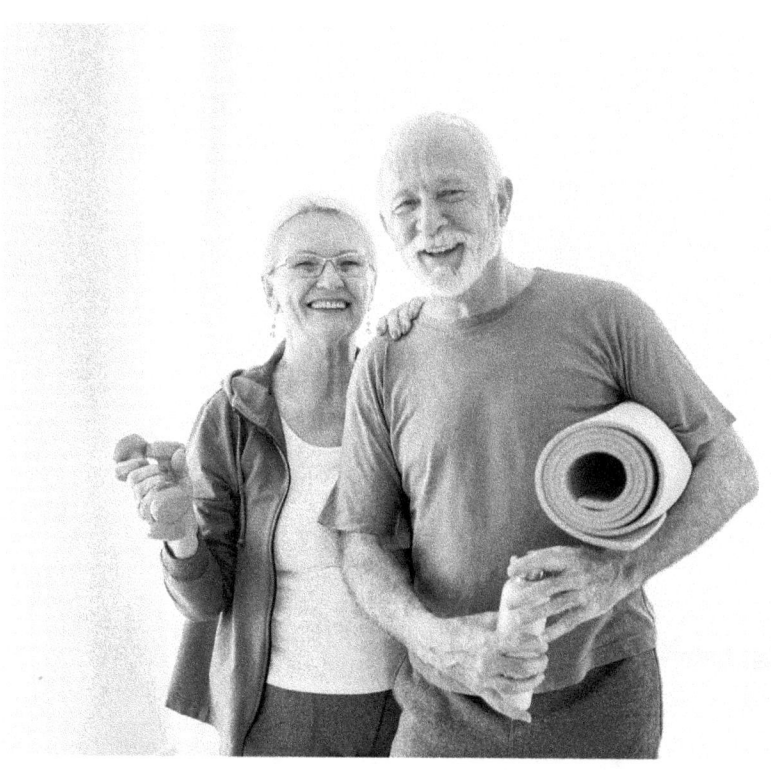

Chapter 6
28-Day Success Plan—Part 1
Days 1-14

Welcome to the 28-Day Success Plan, a carefully crafted journey to immerse you in the transformative world of Wall Pilates. This month-long program is designed to gently guide you through your daily exercises, helping you build strength, flexibility, and confidence. As you start, keep this in mind:

Your plan can take longer than 28 days. As you progress, you may find that starting slower is best for you. Adding additional "rest days" to your routine (days of alternate exercise such as walking, biking, etc.) is ok. The plan is not tagged to specific days of the week, so adding days will not impact the order. Just make sure if you add a rest day that you do not count it as one of the 28 days in the plan. Simply pick up where you left off.

Breath control is important. Focus on exhaling during moments of effort while you exercise. This simple technique aids in effectively engaging your core, providing stability and power to your movements. With each breath, you'll feel more connected to your body and more empowered in your practice. It also helps rid the body of exercise bi-products and brings fresh oxygen to the muscles when they most need it.

Adapt for your level. As you get stronger, you can increase the number of reps for exercises or add simple weights or resistance bands to keep the workouts challenging. Feel free to do so. And, while it's important to challenge yourself, it's equally important to listen to your body. Don't overdo it. Just as you can increase an exercise that's not challenging enough, you can also decrease intensity to prevent overexertion or injury. And while "rest days" are crucial for recovery, keep in mind that consistency is key. By establishing a regular routine, you'll create lasting habits that support your health and vitality and help you meet your goals.

Good posture is not just for exercise time—it's a habit that can enhance your quality of life. Awareness can reinforce the benefits of your Pilates practice and help maintain alignment and balance.

Consider keeping a workout journal to track your progress and reflect on your experiences. Logging the ease or difficulty of each exercise can help tailor upcoming routines to better suit your needs. This journal will become a testament to your dedication and growth over the next 28 days.

How it Works

The 28-Day Plan gets harder as you move through the month. "Rest days" are built-in and are meant to be a break from the direct muscle workouts. During these days, we recommend doing something other than the Wall Pilates routines. For instance, a brisk walk, swimming, biking, or even a few of the breathing routines from the earlier chapters. If you need to change the order or frequency of the rest days, feel free to do so by adding, subtracting, or moving them around, especially in the beginning. For instance, if you need a break after day two instead of day 3, do it! Just pick up where you left off. Also, if you feel you want to shorten a day, that's fine, too.

As you embark on this 28-Day Plan, remember that every day is an opportunity for growth. Celebrate each milestone, stay consistent, and enjoy the journey toward a healthier, more vibrant you.

If you haven't done so yet, be sure to download the free Wall Pilates reference chart. We also have free demonstration videos showing how to properly do the exercises in this book. See Chapter 13 for instructions on how to access these.

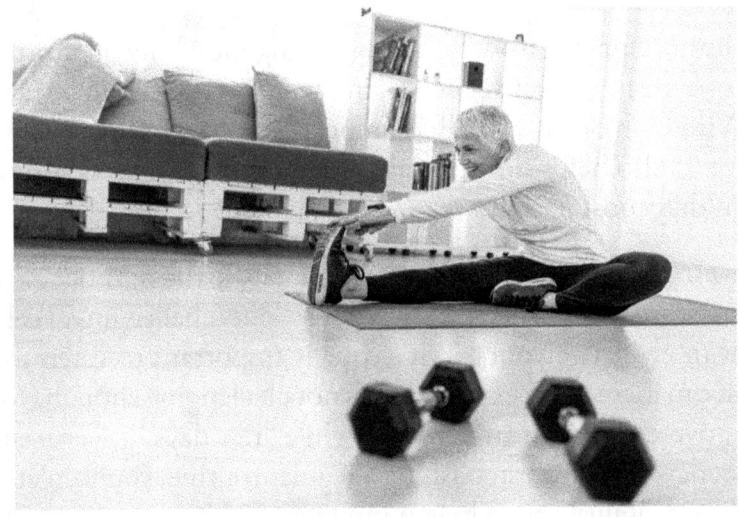

Day 1-Warm-ups first. You'll get used to seeing these stretches!

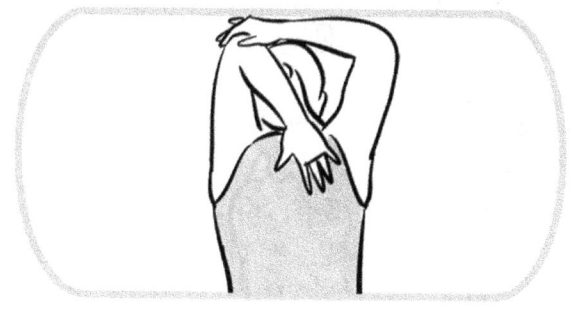

Tricep/Scapula Stretch
Works: Shoulders, Chest, Spine, Back
Benefits: Warm-up & Flexibility

Stand facing away from the wall and raise your left arm overhead. Bend your elbow so your arm is behind your head and your hand is on your upper back. Use your right arm to pull the elbow closer to your head and push down slightly. Allow your muscles to gently release as you hold the stretch for 30 seconds. Repeat with the opposite arm.

Single Arm Pec Stretch
Works: Back, Chest, Shoulders
Benefits: Flexibility, Warm-Up

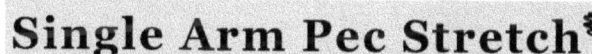
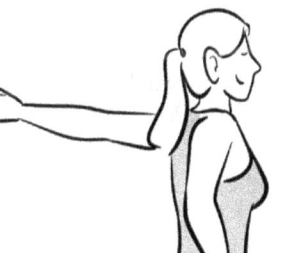
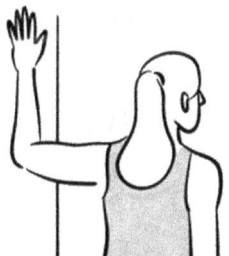

This exercise can be done with your arm extended or bent at the elbow. For arm extended, stand facing the wall an arm's length away. Lift your left arm to shoulder height, place your palm on the wall and twist your body gently to the right. Hold for ten seconds. Focus on feeling a stretch in the chest and shoulders. Repeat the stretch on the opposite side. For bent arm, bend your arm at the elbow.

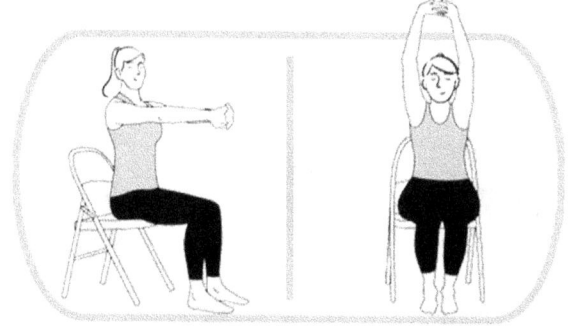

The Scoop
Works: Shoulders, Chest, Spine, Upper Back
Benefits: Posture, Flexibility, Breathing

Interlock your fingers and inhale as you bring them towards your chin. Exhale slowly as you straighten your elbows and turn your interlocked palms outward until your arms are fully extended. Keep the motion going as you raise your hands above your head with your palms towards the ceiling. Release your hands, turn your palms out, and bring them slowly to your sides. Repeat five times.

Arm Raises on the Wall

Works: Back and Spine
Benefits: Posture and Mobility

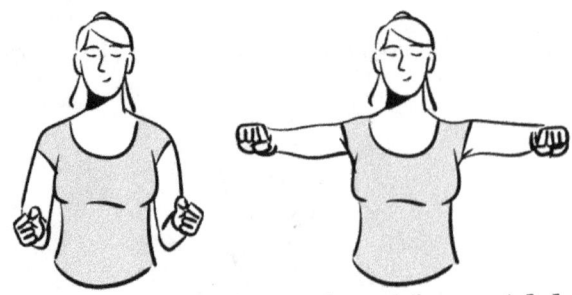

Start with your back against the wall and your feet shoulder-width apart. Spread your arms then bend your elbows so that that your forearms are pointed out in front of you. Keep your upper arms against the wall and raise your elbows up toward the ceiling. Repeat five to ten times.

Wall Angels

Works: Back, Chest, Shoulders
Benefits: Flexibility, Warm-Up

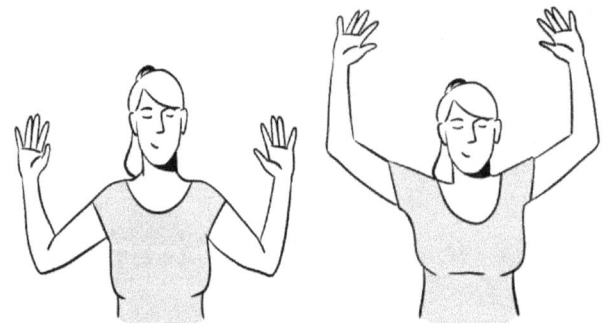

Stand with your back to the wall and feet about six inches away. Bend your arms 90 degrees while keeping them as flat against the wall as possible. From that position, keep your back and arms on the wall and slowly raise your arms up as far as possible. Hold briefly at the top and bring back down to the starting position. Repeat five to ten times.

Large Front Arm Circles

Works: Shoulders, Obliques, Lats
Benefits: Flexibility & Mobility

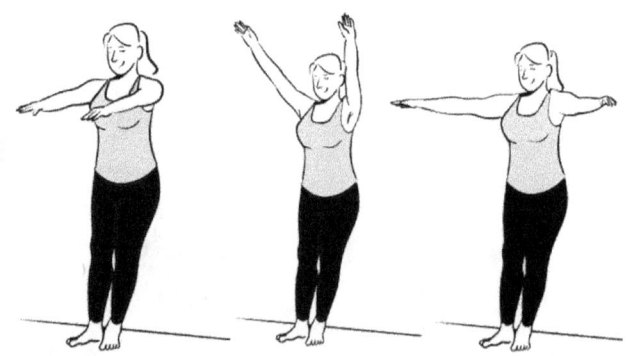

With your back against the wall, bend your knees slightly, raise your arms in front with your elbows locked. Raise them above your head then out to your sides like an airplane and then down. That's one circle. Do ten slow circles in each direction.

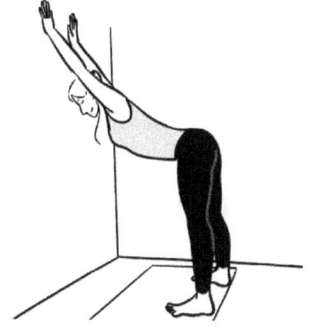

Arms Overhead

Works: Shoulders, Chest, Spine, Back
Benefits: Flexibility & Strength

Stand facing the wall, an arm's length away. Raise your arms over your head and place your palms flat against the wall. Keep your arms straight, lean forward and until you feel a stretch in your upper chest. Hold the stretch for 20-30 seconds, then relax and repeat. For more difficulty, put your palms together as you raise your arms.

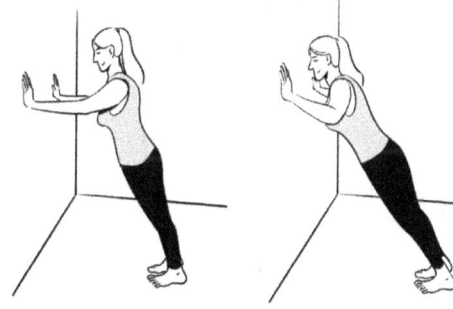

Wall Push-Ups

Works: Back, Chest, Shoulders, Triceps
Benefits: Flexibility, Warm-Up

Stand about an arms' length away and put your palms flat on the wall, about shoulder-width apart. With your arms straight, and your fingers pointing upward, take a small step back, so you are leaning against your hands. Keeping your back straight, slowly bend your arms until your head touches the wall. Pause. Slowly push yourself away from the wall and back up. That's one. Do this 10-15 times.

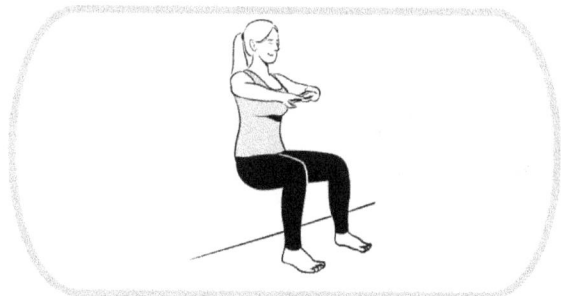

Wall Sit

Works: Quads, Hamstring, Glutes, Core
Benefits: Walking, Climbing, Balance & Coordination

Stand with your back against the wall with your feet shoulder-width apart. Walk your feet out slightly and stretch your arms straight out in front of you as you slowly lower your body down the wall, keeping your feet flat on the floor. Stop when your thighs are parallel to the floor and hold for 30 seconds. Extend your arms in front of you to make it more difficult.

That's it for our first day. See you tomorrow.

Day 2- Let's start with our familiar warm-up stretches.

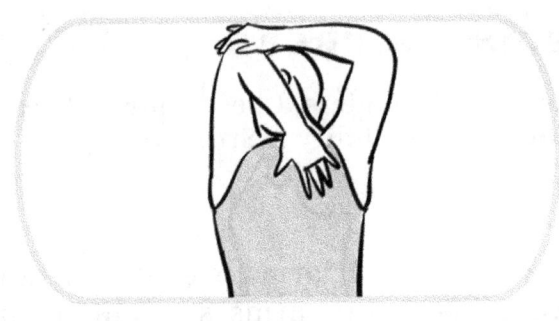

Tricep/Scapula Stretch
Works: Shoulders, Chest, Spine, Back
Benefits: Warm-up & Flexibility

Stand facing away from the wall and raise your left arm overhead. Bend your elbow so your arm is behind your head and your hand is on your upper back. Use your right arm to pull the elbow closer to your head and push down slightly. Allow your muscles to gently release as you hold the stretch for 30 seconds. Repeat with the opposite arm.

Single Arm Pec Stretch
Works: Back, Chest, Shoulders
Benefits: Flexibility, Warm-Up

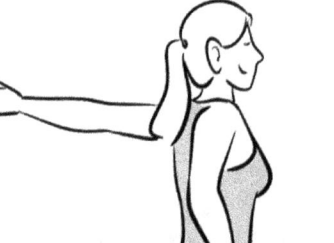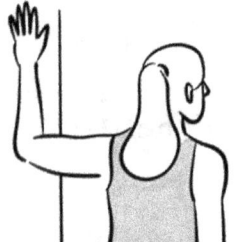

This exercise can be done with your arm extended or bent at the elbow. For arm extended, stand facing the wall an arm's length away. Lift your left arm to shoulder height, place your palm on the wall and twist your body gently to the right. Hold for ten seconds. Focus on feeling a stretch in the chest and shoulders. Repeat the stretch on the opposite side. For bent arm, bend your arm at the elbow.

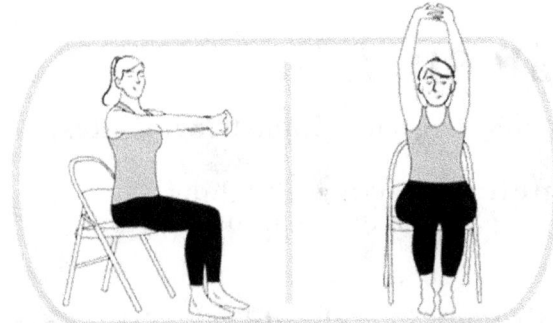

The Scoop
Works: Shoulders, Chest, Spine, Upper Back
Benefits: Posture, Flexibility, Breathing

Interlock your fingers and inhale as you bring them towards your chin. Exhale slowly as you straighten your elbows and turn your interlocked palms outward until your arms are fully extended. Keep the motion going as you raise your hands above your head with your palms towards the ceiling. Release your hands, turn your palms out, and bring them slowly to your sides. Repeat five times.

Now, on to the main routines.

Arm Rolls
Works: Shoulders, Upper Back
Benefits: Flexibility, Strength, Cardio

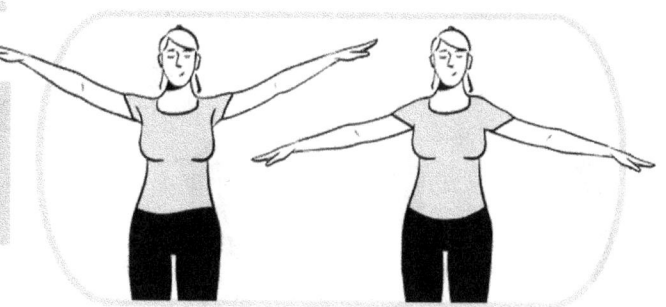

With your back against the wall, or slightly away, bend your knees a bit, bring your arms out to your sides like an airplane, and do ten tight circles in each direction.

Ankle Circles
Works: Ankles, Calves
Benefits: Warm-Up, Stretching

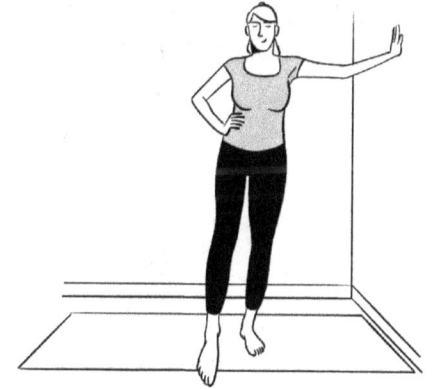

While seated or standing, lift your foot off the floor and slowly make ten circles with your ankles, first in a clockwise direction and then in a counterclockwise direction. Repeat with the opposite foot.

Lateral Leg Swings
Works: Hips, Glutes, Lower Body
Benefits: Flexibility, Mobility, Balance & Strength

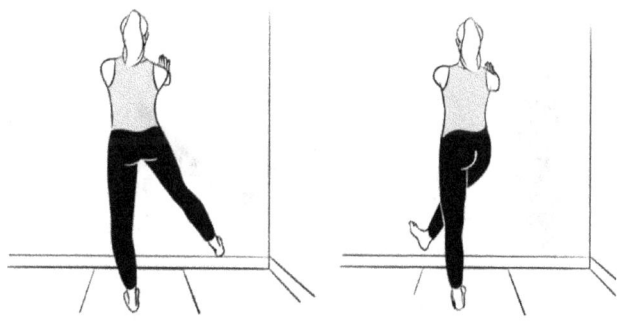

Stand straight with your palms on the wall. Exhale and swing your right leg laterally in front of your left leg towards your left side. Inhale as you return. Do this ten times then repeat with the left leg.

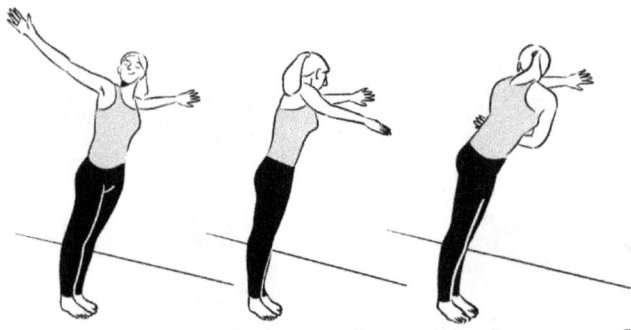

Reach-Twist-Wrap
Works: Legs, Shoulders, Core
Benefits: Balance, Coordination, Strength, Mobility

Start an arm's length away from wall, facing parallel to it. Bend your left arm and place your forearm against the wall. The side of your body should be leaning towards the wall, but straight. Extend your right arm out and slightly up and hold briefly. Twist your body to the left while bringing your right arm down and under the left arm while keeping it away from the body to "wrap" yourself . Inhale as you reach and exhale as you wrap. Repeat 3-5 times each side.

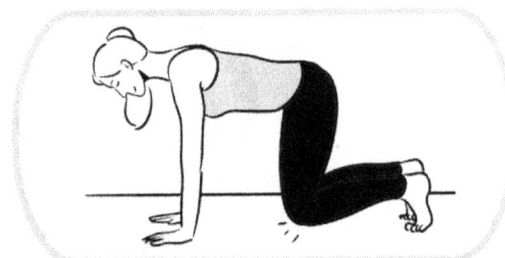

Knee Hover
Works: Core, Hips, Shoulders
Benefits: Stength & Balance

Kneeling on the floor facing the mat with your back straight and your toes on the floor, pick both knees up off the floor about one inch and hold for 30 seconds. Breathe deeply and slowly, and try not to move any other part of your body. Repeat five times.

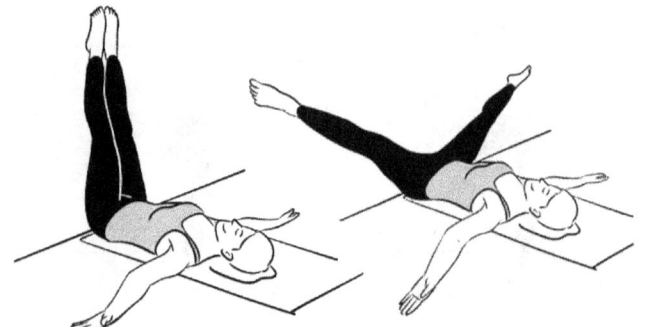

Wall Scissors
Works: Abs, Glutes, Inner Thighs
Benefits: Strength, Coordination, Balance

Lay on your back with your legs bent and your legs and buttocks are against the wall. Stretch your arms out from your side and open your legs widely to stretch the inner thigh and hold for two seconds. Bring back to neutral. Repeat 10 times.

Wall Oblique Twist
Works: Upper Lats, Abs
Benefits: Flexibility, Strength, Mobility

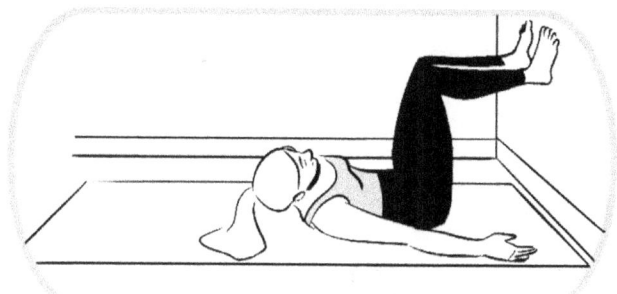

Lie on your back with your hands at your sides, your feet on the wall and your knees bent to form a 90-degre angle. Keeping your arms near the floor, lift your head and neck slightly, bend them to the right as you reach your right hand towards the wall without arching your back. Hold for three seconds and return to neutral position. Repeat on the left side.

Sit Stretch
Works: Ankles, Calves
Benefits: Warm-Up, Stretching

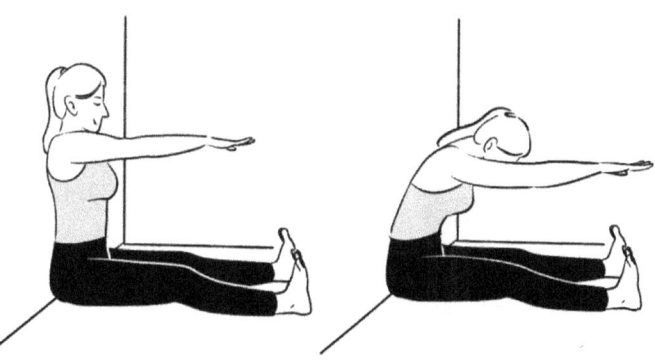

Sit on the floor with your back touching the wall and your arms out in front of you. Slowly bend forward at the waist, so that your is face pointed at the floor. Go as far as you can without straining and hold for 30 seconds. Repeat.

End of Day 2

Day 3

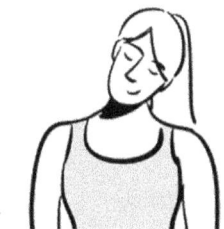 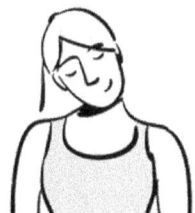

Neck Circles
Works: Neck & Shoulders
Benefits: Warm-Up, Stretch Tension Release

Stand slightly away from the wall with your arms at your sides. Make slow, wide circles with your head; five times clockwise then five times counterclockwise. Concentrate on deep breathing as you do the movement.

Day 3

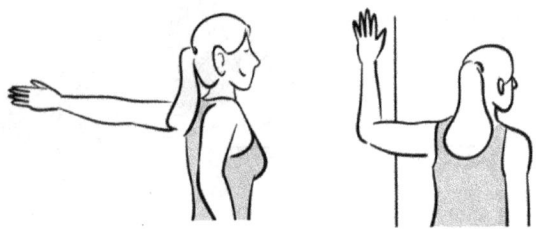

Pec Stretch
Works: Back, Chest, Shoulders
Benefits: Flexibility, Warm-Up

This exercise can be done with your arm extended or bent at the elbow. For arm extended, stand facing the wall an arm's length away. Lift your left arm to shoulder height, place your palm on the wall and twist your body gently to the right. Hold for ten seconds. Focus on feeling a stretch in the chest and shoulders. Repeat the stretch on the opposite side. For bent arm, bend your arm at the elbow.

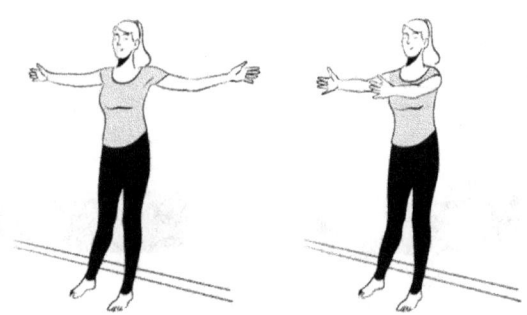

Bird Flap
Works: Scapula, Chest, Shoulders
Benefits: Flexibility, Balance

Stand with your back to the wall, with your feet two feet away. Spread your arms like an airplane, with the backs of your arms touching the wall and your palms facing out. Keeping your elbows locked, bring your arms straight out in front of you so that your thumbs are up and your palms are facing each other and nearly touching. Hold briefly and return. That's one. Repeat at a medium speed 15 times.

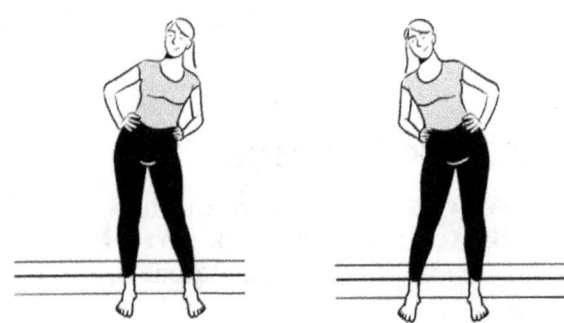

Large Hip Circles
Works: Hips, Upper Legs
Benefits: Flexibility, Mobility, Balance, Strength

Stand facing the wall, with your feet shoulder-width apart about two feet from the wall. Put your hands on the hips and pull your abs in to engage your core muscles. Bend to the side slightly and rotate your hips clockwise 10 times at a medium speed. Repeat in the other direction. Increase the size of the circles as you become more flexible and comfortable with the exercise.

Day 3

Wall Russian Twists
Works: Abs, Obliques, Spine
Benefits: Cardio, Strength, Calorie Burn

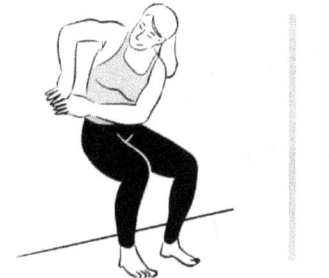
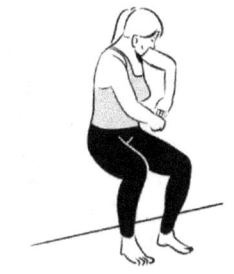

Stand with your knees bent and your back against the wall in as simi-squat position. Quickly twist your torso to the left while reaching your right arm across your body to touch the wall on your left with your right hand. Twist your torso back to the right while reaching your left arm across your body to touch the wall on your right with your left hand. Repeat this side-to-side motion 20 times for two sets.

Side Plank
Works: Obliques, Core
Benefits: Strength, Stability, Balance

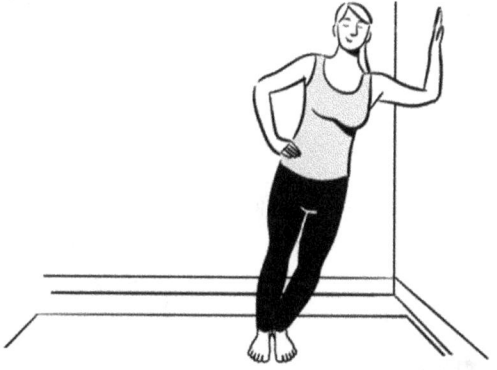

Stand next to the wall, about three feet away. Keep your body straight and lean sideways with your left forearm on the wall to support your body. Hold for 30 to 60 seconds and then change sides for a total of two times on each side.

Torso Twist on Mat
Works: Spine, Abs
Benefits: Strength & Mobility

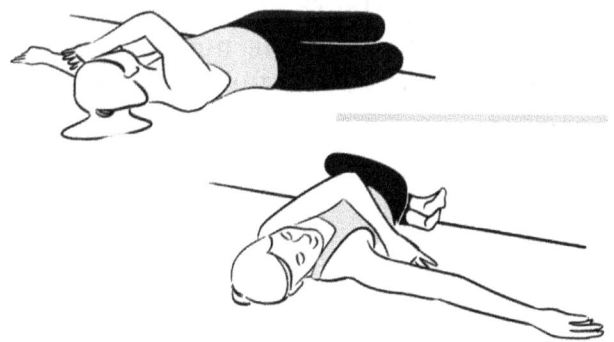

Lie on your back with your feet touching the wall. Rotate your arms, torso and head to your left while rotating your legs to the right. Keep your abs tight to avoid straining your lower back. Repeat the motion on the right side. That is one repetition. Do ten medium-speed reps.

Day 3

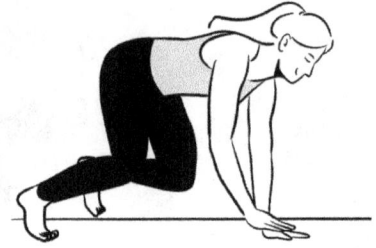

Balance Bear
Works: Arms, Shoulders, Core.
Benefits: Strength, Stability, Balance

Start on your hands and knees with your hands under your shoulders and your legs bent so that your knees are under your hips. Lift your knees off the floor so your shins are parallel with it. Keeping your back straight, lift your right hand and your left foot about an inch, then replace, then lift your left hand and your right foot about an inch and then replace. That's one repetition. Do a total of ten reps, rest for 30 seconds, and then repeat once more.

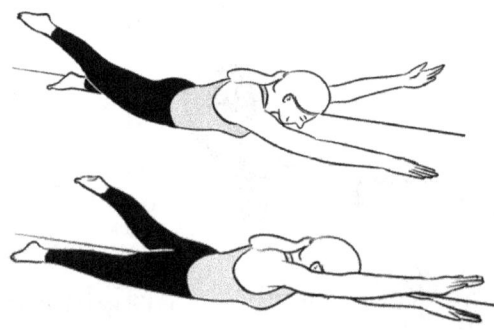

Swimmer's Reach
Works: Abs, Back, Shoulders, Hips
Benefits: Flexibility & Mobility

Laying face-down on a mat parallel to the wall, stretch out your legs behind you and your arms above your head with palms on the mat. Your head can be up or resting on the mat. Breathe in and raise your locked right arm and left leg straight up at the same time, keeping them parallel to the floor. Hold momentarily and breathe out as you return them to the mat. Repeat with the left arm and the right leg. That's one repetition. Repeat for a total of ten repetitions.

Congratulations! You've completed the exercises for Day 3.

Day 4: Other Movement & Breathing

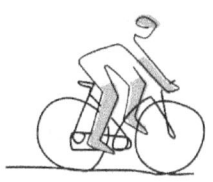 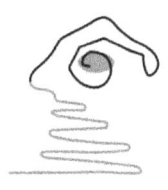 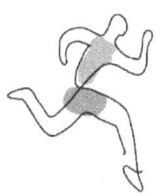 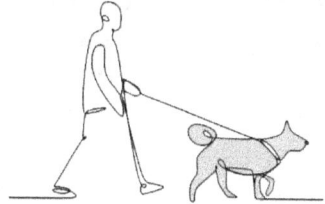

On this "rest" day, enjoy an alternate exercise such as brisk walking, swimming, or biking. Or try a few of the following breathing exercises. Find a quiet place where you can concentrate and feel free to play some relaxing music while you're doing these. (There are no illustrations for the breathing exercises).

Belly Breathing
Benefit: Breath Control
Instructions: To start, sit comfortably with your back straight. Put one hand on your chest and the other on your belly. Breathe in deeply through the nose, allowing your belly to expand while keeping your chest still. Hold momentarily and then exhale slowly through your mouth, drawing your belly inward. Breathe in, breathe out. Pay specific attention to your belly's rise and fall. Once again: breathe in, breathe out. Continue for three to five minutes.

Ocean Sounding Breath
Benefit: Concentration
Instructions: This exercise adds a bit of complexity by involving your throat and is great for relaxation and clearing your head. To begin, sit upright with your shoulders relaxed. Slowly inhale through your nose. Exhale through your mouth while slightly constricting the back of the throat, producing a soft sound like you're fogging a pane of glass or a mirror. Try to make this soft sound while inhaling and exhaling. Once again: inhale through the nose, and then exhale through the mouth making the fogging sound. Repeat ten times.

Box Breathing
Benefits: Stress Relief & Discipline
Instructions: Inhale through the nose slowly while counting to four in your head. Hold that breath for a count of four. Exhale through your mouth for a count of four. Hold that breath out for another count of four. Complete 5-10 cycles.

Nostril Yoga Breathing
Benefits: Calming and Stress Relief
Instructions: Start by closing your right nostril with your right thumb and inhaling through your left nostril. Next, close your left nostril with your ring finger, releasing your right nostril. Exhale through the right nostril. Inhale through the right nostril, close it with your right thumb, then exhale through the left nostril. This is one cycle. Complete four cycles.

Hissing Breath
Benefit: Concentration
Instructions: The "hissing" serves as a focal point, making it easier to concentrate on the breath and clear the mind. To start, inhale deeply through the nose and then exhale slowly through clenched teeth, creating a hissing sound as the air escapes. Repeat five to ten times.

Humming Breath
Benefit: Concentration
Instructions: Start by finding a comfortable but upright position in your chair. Close your eyes and take a slow, deep breath through your nose. Exhale slowly through your mouth while producing a humming sound. Repeat ten times.

Cooling Breath
Benefit: Concentration & Physical Cooling
Instructions: This technique has a calming effect on the nervous system and can purportedly cool down the body. This can be particularly effective on hot days or after a series of vigorous exercises. To begin, sit upright, making sure your posture is open but relaxed. Stick your tongue out and roll it like a tube. Inhale through this tubular tongue.... Close your mouth and exhale normally through the nose. Repeat ten cycles.

Incorporating these stand-alone breathing exercises into your day and routines can significantly enhance your overall energy and concentration and help you experience a renewed sense of vitality extending far beyond your workout sessions.

This marks the end of Day 4.

Day 5. Let's start with a few warm-ups.

Single Arm Pec Stretch

Works: Back, Chest, Shoulders
Benefits: Flexibility, Warm-Up

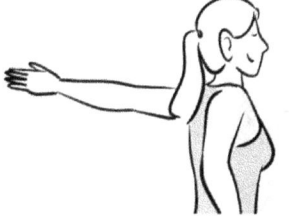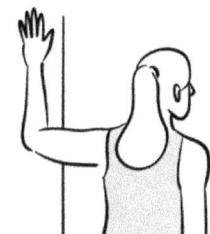

This exercise can be done with your arm extended or bent at the elbow. For arm extended, stand facing the wall an arm's length away. Lift your left arm to shoulder height, place your palm on the wall and twist your body gently to the right. Hold for ten seconds. Focus on feeling a stretch in the chest and shoulders. Repeat the stretch on the opposite side. For bent arm, bend your arm at the elbow.

The Scoop

Works: Shoulders, Chest, Spine, Upper Back
Benefits: Posture, Flexibility, Breathing

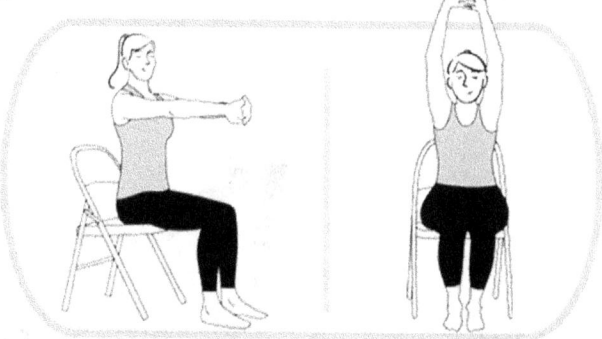

Interlock your fingers and inhale as you bring them towards your chin. Exhale slowly as you straighten your elbows and turn your interlocked palms outward until your arms are fully extended. Keep the motion going as you raise your hands above your head with your palms towards the ceiling. Release your hands, turn your palms out and bring them slowly to your sides. Repeat five times.

Arm Rolls

Works: Shoulders, Back
Benefits: Flexibility, Cardio

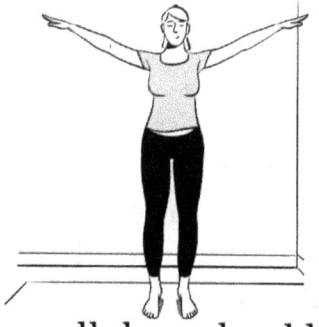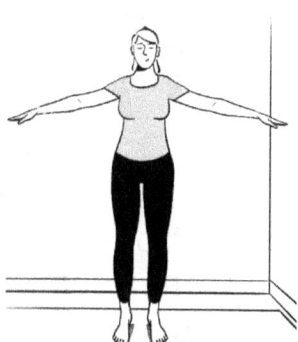

Stand about three feet from the wall, legs shoulder length apart and your arms out like an airplane. Keeping your elbows locked, make large, forward circles with your arms at medium speed. Do this five times then switch directions for five more repetitions. Repeat in each direction five times.

Day 5 Main Exercises

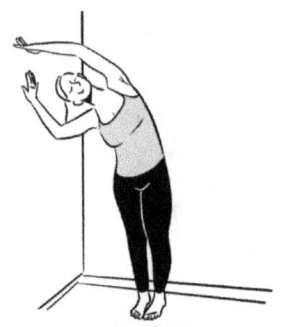

Side Bend

Works: Obliques, Inner Thigh, Glutes, Hips, Core
Benefits: Balance, Flexibility

Begin by standing sideways and an arm's length from the wall, with your right side closest to the wall and feet hip-width apart. Put your right palm on the wall, extend your left arm overhead, and slide your right hand down the wall as you bend your torso to the right and touch the wall.

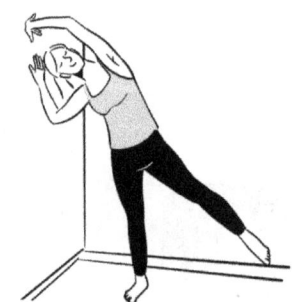

Side Bend & Leg Lifts

Works: Obliques, Inner Thigh, Glutes, Hips, Core
Benefits: Balance, Flexibility

Hold the "Side Bend" position of the previous exercise, while lifting your left leg up and out sideways for ten repetitions. Return to start, then switch sides and repeat. Do this twice for each leg.

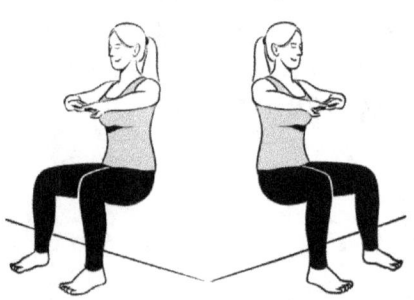

Wall Sit

Works: Quads, Hamstrings, Glutes
Benefits: Walking, Climbing, Balance, Coordination

This exercise predominantly works the quadriceps (the four muscles at the front of the thigh) important for knee stability, walking, getting up from a seated position, and climbing. To begin, stand with your back against the wall with your feet shoulder-width apart. Walk your feet out slightly so that your back is leaning against the wall slightly. Slowly lower your body down the wall, keeping your feet flat on the floor. Stop when your thighs are parallel to the floor. Hold for 30 seconds. Extend your arms out to make it harder.

Day 5

Bear Walk: Fwd & Back
Works: Arms, Shoulders, Calves, Core
Benefits: Balance, Stretgth, Mobility

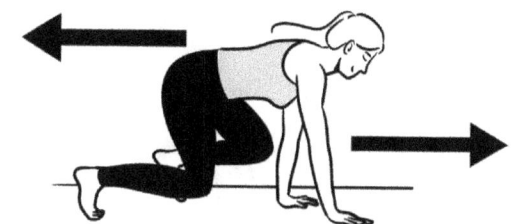

Start on all fours (hands and feet) with your shins parallel with the floor. From this position, lift your right hand and left foot, and take a step forward, keeping your back straight. Continue this walking motion for about 10 steps, pausing between steps and alternating feet and hands each time. Then reverse direction by walking in the same manner backwards to your starting spot. Do five repetitions of this back and forth walk.

Bear Walk: Sideways
Works: Arms, Shoulders, Calves, Core
Benefits: Balance, Stretgth, Mobility

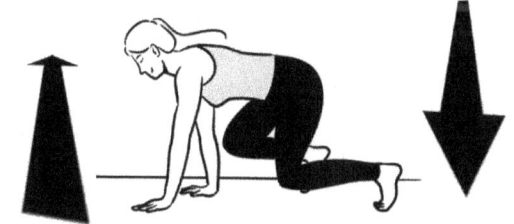

This is the "Bear Walk" to the sides. Start in a Balance Bear Pose:on all fours (hands and feet) with your shins parallel to the floor and your back straight. From this position, lift your right hand and left foot, and take a step sideways, keeping your back straight. Continue this walking motion for about 10 steps, then reverse direction by walking in the same manner to your starting spot. Do five reps of this back and forth walk.

Wall Bicycle Crunch
Works: Abs, Love Handles
Benefits: Strength & Cardio

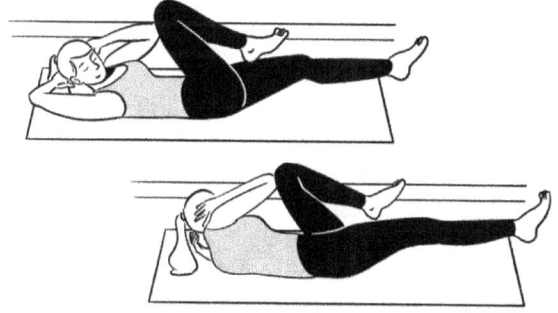

Lie on your back with your feet on the wall and your hands behind your head. To start, bring your right knee up as you bend your left elbow down to touch it. Then cross to the opposite side by bringing your left knee up as you bend to touch your right elbow to meet it. That's one. Aim for 10-20 repetitions and two sets.

Day 5

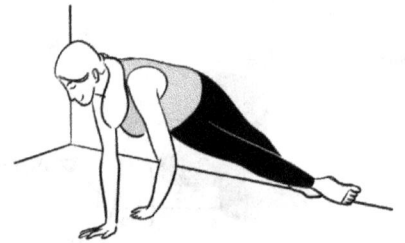

Thread the Needle
Works: Arms, Chest, Core
Benefits: Crdo, Strength, Flexibility

Start on your belly in the push-up position. Place your feet in the crevice between the wall and floor with your left toes touching your right heel. Lift your left arm to the ceiling and then rotate your torso to bring your left arm slowly back down between your chest and the floor. Repeat five times then switch sides.

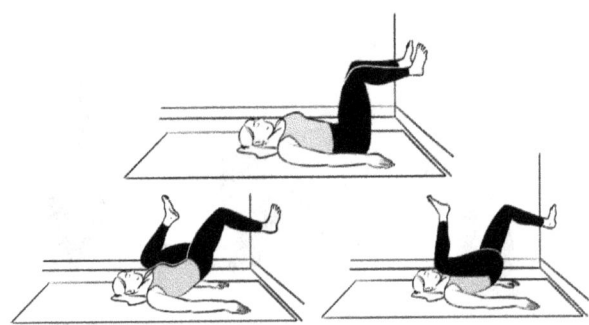

Knee Tucks to Chest
Works: Obliques, Hamstrings, Glutes, Hips, Core
Benefits: Balance, Flexibility, Mobility

Lay flat on your back and place your knees at a 90° angle against the wall. Extend your arms along your sides. Use your left leg to give a push towards your chest, lifting your hips (the knee will be towards the chest). Repeat the same movement with your right leg. Avoid arching your back and inhale as you give the push and exhale as you bring your foot towards the wall. Repeat ten times.

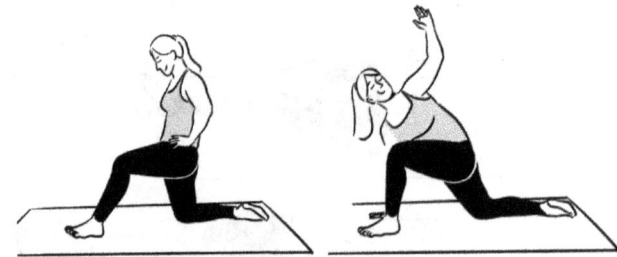

Multi-Stretch Move
Works: Hamstrings, Glutes, Hip Flexors, Obliques
Benefits: Walking, Climbing, Balance, Coordination

Start on your knees parallel to the wall. Stretch your left leg out in front of you with your leg bent and the foot flat on the floor. Lean forward with your torso to add a stretch to the planted knee's hip flexor. Place one hand on the floor opposite to the front foot. Finally, reach your left arm up and rotate towards the ceiling leading with your upper back and shoulders. Hold for 3 seconds then repeat on the opposite side.

This concludes the exercises for Day 5.

Day 6 starts with a few of our familiar warm-up moves.

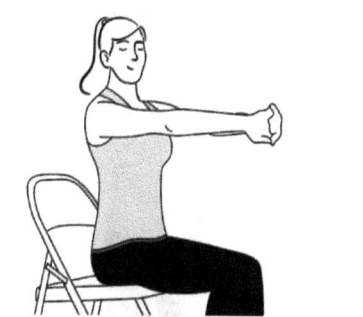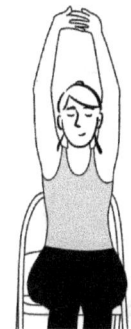

Scoop

Works: Shoulders, Chest, Spine
Benefits: Posture, flexibility, Breathing

Interlock your fingers and inhale as you bring them towards your chin. Exhale as you straighten your elbows and turn your interlocked palms outward until your arms are fully extended. Keep the motion going as you raise your hands above your head with your palms towards the ceiling. Release your hands, turn your palms out, and bring them slowly to your sides. Repeat five times.

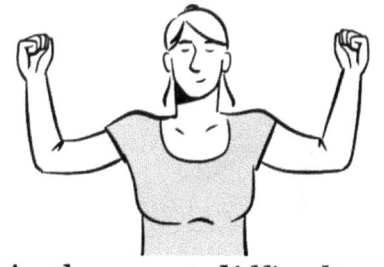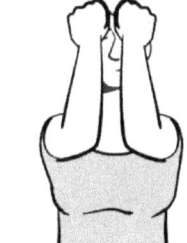

Cactus Arms

Works: Back, Chest, Spine, Shoulders
Benefits: Warm-Up & Flexibility

The starting position of this one is the most difficult, especially if you sit at a desk for long stretches. This will get easier as you practice and stretch out the muscles and associated tendons and ligaments in the back, chest, and shoulders. Start with your back and body against the wall and your arms bent up at the elbow at a 90-degree angle like a cactus. Move your arms forward so that your palms and forearms come together in front of you. Pause briefly. With your elbows still bent, move your arms back so that the back of your hands and forearms touch the wall. Hold briefly. Repeat 10 times.

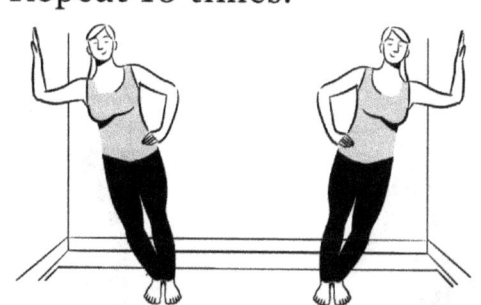

Side Plank

Works: Obliques, Core
Benefits: Strength, Stability, Balance

Stand next to the wall and about three feet away. Put your right hand on your right hip and bend your left elbow in a 90-degree angle. Keep your body straight and lean sideways, placing your left forearm on the wall so it's supporting you on the wall. Hold for 30-60 seconds on each side. Repeat two times on each side.

Day 6 Main Exercises

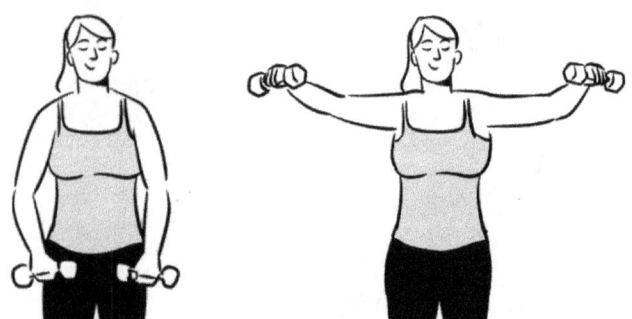

Lateral Raises
Works: Deltoids, Upper Back
Benefits: Cardio & Strength

Start with empty hands and add weights or bands as it gets easier. To Start, stand upright with your arms bent at the elbows. Bring both elbows straight up to shoulder level as if pouring water out of a pitcher. Bring back to start and repeat. Do this 6-10 times. Increase weight as you get stronger.

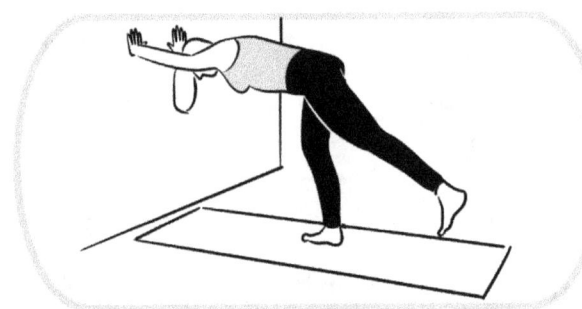

Rear Leg Lifts
Works: Hamstrings, Glutes, Groin
Benefits: Cardio. Stability, Balance

Start by facing the wall a bit more than an arm's length away. Bend at the waist keeping your body straight and put your palms on the wall bending until your body forms an "L". Keeping your hips pointing towards the floor, swing your right leg out behind you and up as far as you comfortably can. Hold for 1 second and bring back to the start position. That's one. Repeat for a total of ten repetitions then switch to the left leg for ten reps.

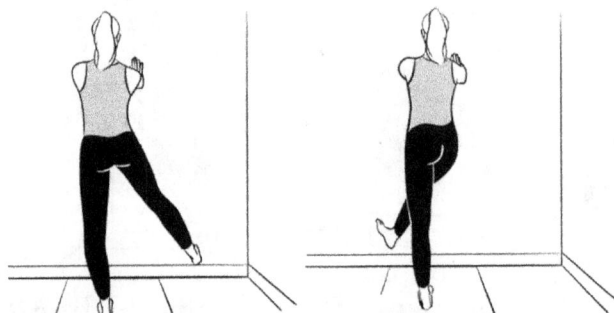

Inner Thigh Leg Lifts
Works: Glutes, Hips, Groin
Benefits: Strength, Stability, Balance

Face the wall about 3-4 feet away. Lean over and put your palms on the wall. Keeping your back and spine straight, swing your left leg in front of and across your body to the right side and back. That's one. Repeat ten times then switch sides.

Day 6

Knee Extension

Works: Upper Lats, Quads,. Glutes
Benefits: Strength, Stability, Balance

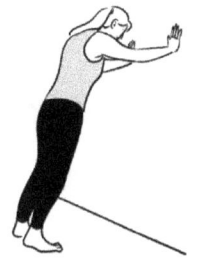 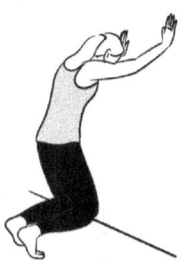

Start by facing the wall about one and a half arm's lengths away. Lean over and place your hands on the wall without bending your knees. Keep your feet in place and slowly bend at the knees towards the wall. Hold momentarily before coming back to the starting position. Do this 10 times.

Knee Raises

Works: Core, Hip Flexors, Obliques
Benefits: Stability, Balance, Cardio

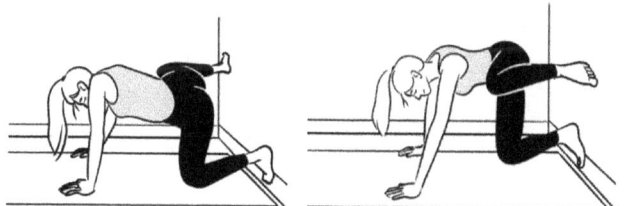

Get on your hands and knees with your toes an inch from the wall behind you. Keeping your back and arms straight and knee bent, spread your legs apart by lifting your bent right leg out and up towards the ceiling Hold momentarily and then back to the floor for 10 times each side.

Hip Flexor Stretch

Works: Hips, Back, Quads, Core   **Benefits:** Balance, Mobility, Flexibility

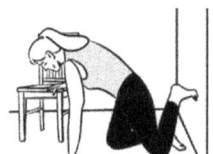 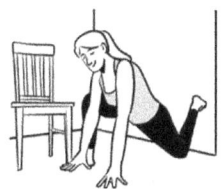 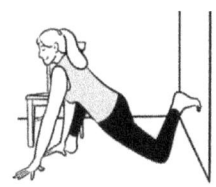 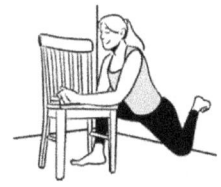

With a chair sideways in front of you, kneel down with your back to and your feet touching the wall. Lean forward so your right hand is on the chair seat for support and your left hand is on the floor. Place your left foot on the wall so that the toes are curled under with the ball of your foot touching. While supporting yourself with the chair, bring your right foot forward and bend your knee so that the foot is flat on the floor. Next, put your right hand on the floor and push your pelvis forward and away from the wall to feel the stretch. Hold for 3-5 seconds and then slightly twist your hips and pelvis to the right as you lift your head. Hold until you feel the muscles loosen (about 10 seconds). Unwind and repeat with the opposite leg on the wall.

Day 6

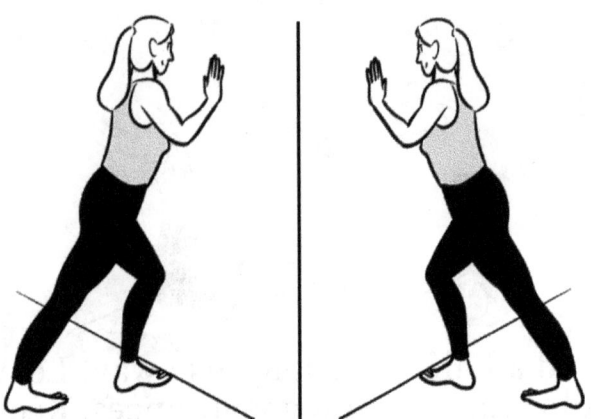

Calf Stretch
Works: Ankle, Quadriceps, Calf
Benefits: Stability, Balance

Stand facing the wall about 1 1/2 arm's lengths away, feet shoulder length apart. Lean forward to the wall, bend your left knee as you slide your right foot back, keeping your foot flat on the floor until you feel the stretch in your calf. Hold for 10 seconds and release. Return to the neutral position and repeat with the opposite leg and calf. An alternate method is to use a stair to stretch, hanging your foot half way off of a step, allowing the heel to drop below the stair to stretch the calf.

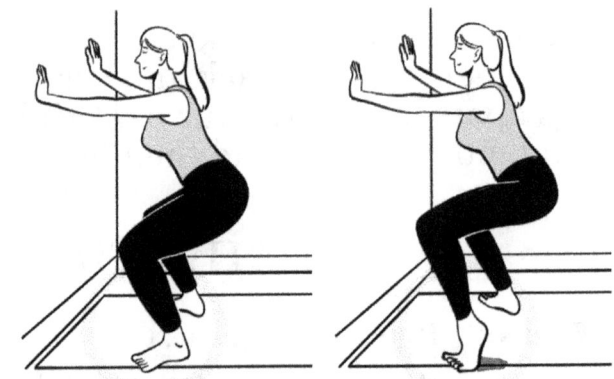

Calf Raise
Works: Ankle, Quadriceps, Calf
Benefits: Stability, Balance

Stand facing the wall, arm's length away with your palms on the wall and feet wide apart. Turn your toes outward and bend your knees to lower down to a 90-degree angle at the knees. Alternate raising your heels off the floor: right-left-right-left. Do 15-20 right-left repetitions then return to starting position.

That's it for your Day 6 exercises. See you tomorrow!

For Day 7, let's start with a few of our familiar warm-up moves.

Tricep/Scapula Stretch
Works: Shoulders, Chest, Spine, Back
Benefits: Warm-up & Flexibility

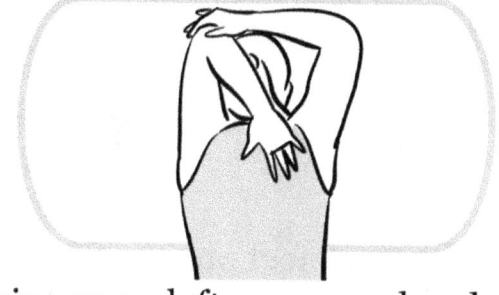

Stand facing away from the wall and raise your left arm overhead. Bend your elbow so your arm is behind your head and your hand is on your upper back. Use your right arm to pull the elbow closer to your head and push down slightly. Allow your muscles to gently release as you hold the stretch for 30 seconds. Repeat with the opposite arm.

Single Arm Pec Stretch
Works: Back, Chest, Shoulders
Benefits: Flexibility, Warm-Up

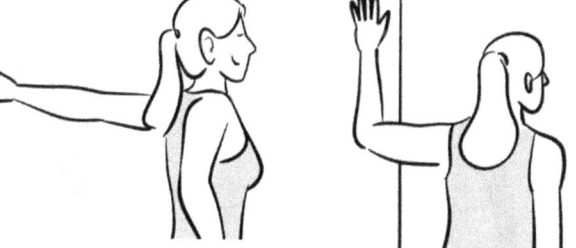

This exercise can be done with your arm extended or bent at the elbow. For arm extended, stand facing the wall an arm's length away. Lift your left arm to shoulder height, place your palm on the wall and twist your body gently to the right. Hold for ten seconds. Focus on feeling a stretch in the chest and shoulders. Repeat the stretch on the opposite side. For bent arm, bend your arm at the elbow.

The Scoop
Works: Shoulders, Chest, Spine, Back
Benefits: Posture, Flexibility, Breathing

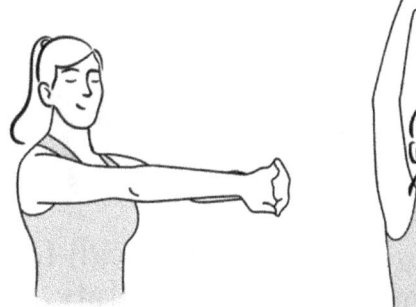
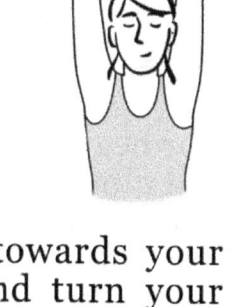

Interlock your fingers and inhale as you bring them towards your chin. Exhale slowly as you straighten your elbows and turn your interlocked palms outward until your arms are fully extended. Keep the motion going as you raise your hands above your head with your palms towards the ceiling. Release your hands, turn your palms out, and bring them slowly to your sides. Repeat five times.

Day 7 Main Exercises

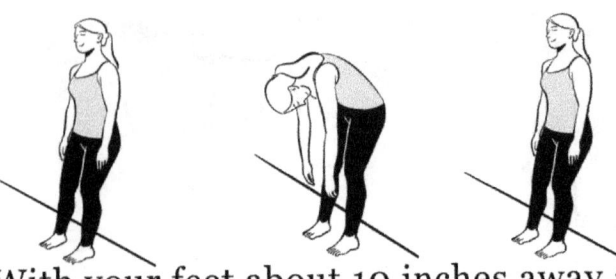

Wall Roll-Down
Works: Abs, Spine
Benefits: Balance, Flexibility

With your feet about 10 inches away and your knees locked, place your back against the wall making sure the area from your head to your hips is on the wall. Keep your back straight, tighten your core, and keep both hands at your sides. Inhale deeply and as you exhale, tuck your chin and slowly rotate your spine from vertebra to vertebra, lowering your upper body as far as your flexibility allows. Return to the starting position by reversing the movement. Inhale, exhale.

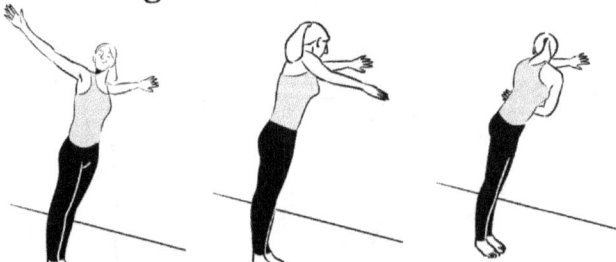

Reach-Twist-Wrap
Works: Legs, Shoulders, Core
Benefits: Balance, coordination, strength, mobility

Start an arm's length away from wall, facing parallel to wall. Bend your left arm and place forearm against wall. Extend your right arm out and slightly up and hold briefly. Twist your body to the left while bringing your right arm down and under the left arm "wrap" your body. Repeat 3-5 times and then switch sides.

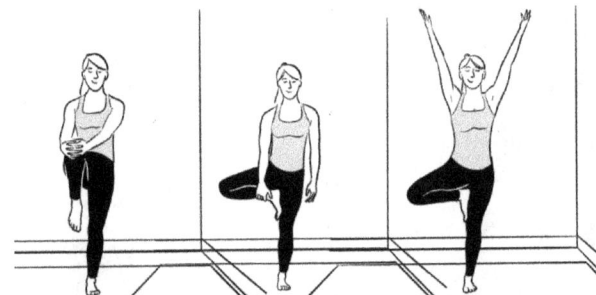

Wall Tree
Works: Legs, Shoulders, Pelvis
Benefits: Balance, Coordination, Flexibility, Pelvic Stability

For beginners, use the wall for balance. Later, do it away from the wall but close enough for safety. Stand facing away from the wall slightly and bend your right knee, grabbing it with your hands and locking them around it. Pause until you are stable and then grab your right foot with your right hand, twisting it slightly so that the inner thigh is looking upward. Bring it up slowly-as high as you can against your left leg with the bottom of your right foot against the side of your left leg. Lock it in if possible then swing your arms up over your head. Hold for 30-60 seconds and then release. Repeat with the left leg.

Day 7

Single Leg Circles
Works: Glutes, Hips, Groin
Benefits: Strength, Stability, Balance

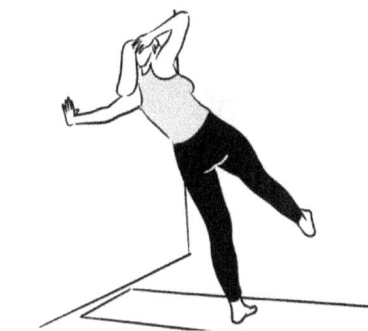

Bend slightly at the hips and place your left hand on the wall. Bend your right elbow and place your right hand on the back of your head. Keeping your left leg straight, make five wide circles with your right leg while keeping your knees locked. Repeat five times in each direction then switch legs.

Press Lunge
Works: Glutes, Hips, Quads, Ankles
Benefits: Flexibility, Mobility, Balance

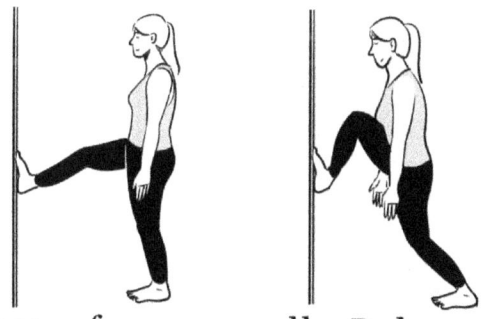

Begin by standing one leg-length away from a wall. Balance yourself, then place one foot on the wall at hip-height. Bend your knee and lunge forward until your quad is in line with your core, keeping your torso neutral and upright. Pause for 1 Second, then press through the ball of your foot to return to your starting position. Repeat the process for each set.

Mountain Climber
Works: Core, Abs, Hips
Benefits: Cardio, Strength, Mobility

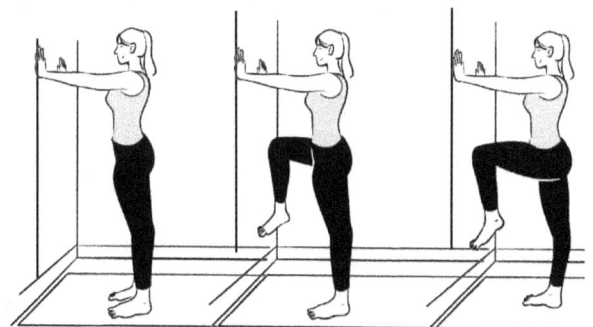

Stand an arm's length away with your palms on the wall in front of you and your arms fully extended but not bent. Bend your leg and lift your right knee towards the wall with your toes and lower leg pointed down. Immediately return to start and repeat with the left leg, while keeping your back straight. The movements should be controlled, but quick. Repeat the back-and-forth motion for 15 reps.

Day 7

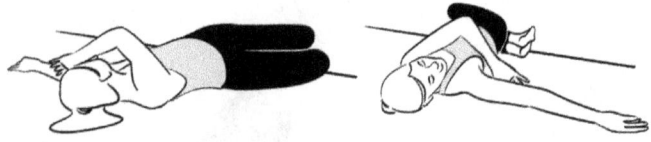

Torso Twist on Mat
Works: Spine, Shoulders, Back
Benefits: Mobility, Flexibility

Lie on your back with your feet touching the wall for reference. Bend your legs at the knees slightly and rotate them to the right so your knees touch the mat. At the same time, extend your arms across your torso to the left, trying to touch the mat on the left side. Hold for three to five seconds and repeat on the opposite sides.

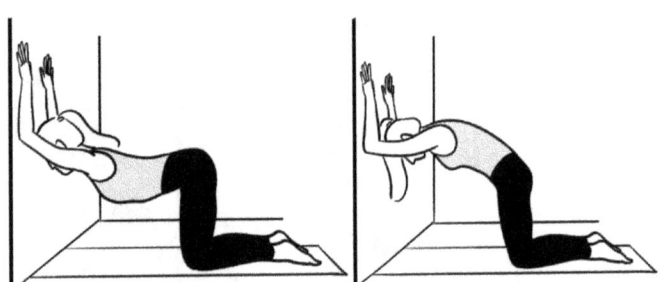

Cat-Cow
Works: Spine, Shoulders, Back
Benefits: Mobility, Flexibility

Get on your hands and knees facing the wall about an arm's length away. Lean into the wall and put your elbows, forearms and palms on the wall while arching your back. Hold for three seconds while inhaling and exhaling, then roll your back down while sticking your buttocks out. your back should now be in a simi "U" shape. Hold for five seconds while you inhale and exhale then return.

This marks the end of "Day 7" exercises.

Day 8: Alternate Exercises & Rest

Today you can take a rest from Wall Pilates and enjoy an alternate exercise on your own such as brisk walking, swimming, or biking. You can also do some of the simple stretching and breathing exercises from earlier chapters in the book.

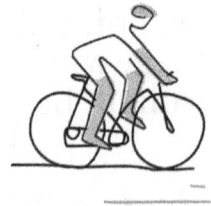 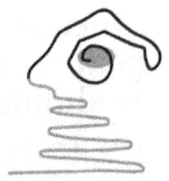 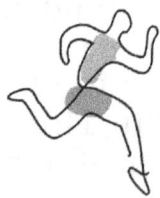 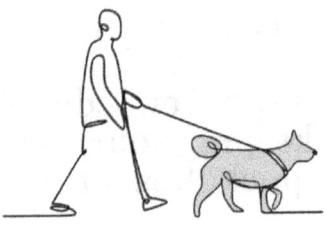

Day 9. Let's jump right in with our warm-ups.

Arm Slides
Works: Core, Legs, Shoulders
Benefits: Cardio, Mobility, Warm-Up

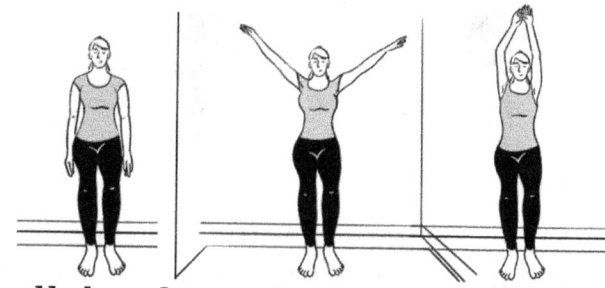

Standing with your back to the wall, bend your knees as you walk your feet out about an arm's length out in front of you while keeping your back and buttocks on the wall into a partial wall sit position. Keeping your elbows locked, slide your arms straight up above your head until your hands meet. Hold momentarily and then bring them back down. That's one. Repeat for ten total.

Ankle Circles
Works: Ankles, Calves
Benefits: Balance, Mobility. Warm-Up

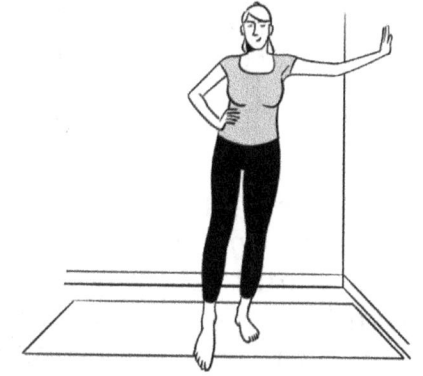

While seated or standing with your feet up, make five clockwise circles with your right foot, centered on the ankle, then five in a counter-clockwise direction. Switch to the left foot and repeat.

Calf Stretch
Works: Calf, Ankles
Benefits: Leg Strength & Warm-Up

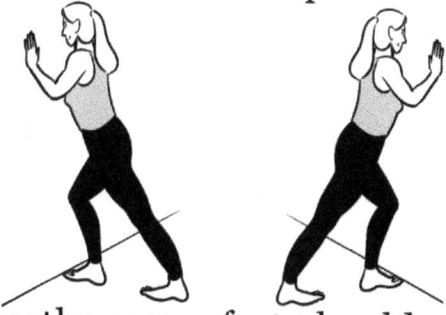

Stand facing the wall about 1 1/2 arms lengths away, feet shoulder length apart. Lean forward to the wall, bend your left knee as you slide the right foot back, keeping your right foot flat on the floor until you feel the stretch in your right calf. Hold for 10 seconds then point your right toe outward continuing the stretch for 10 more seconds. Next, point your right toe inward to stretch for another 10 seconds. Return to neutral position and repeat with the opposite leg and calf.

Day 9

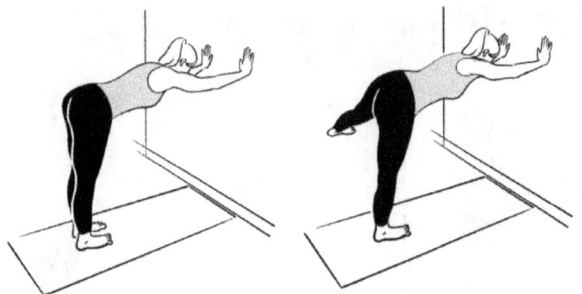

Fwd Bend Side Leg Lift
Works: Inner Thigh, Hips, Core
Benefits: Balance, Mobility, Cardio

Stand facing the wall and bend forward until your torso is parallel to the floor, your arms straight, and your palms flat against the wall. Lift your left leg out to the side until it's parallel to the floor (or as high as you can), keeping your hips level. Do 10 repetitions and repeat with the right leg. You can also alternate between legs (left-right) for 20 reps and more of a cardio action.

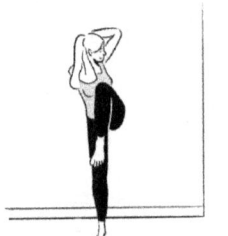 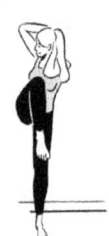

Standing Bicycle
Works: Back, Spine, Hip Flexors, Abs
Benefits: Cardio, Strength, Balance, Mobility

Lean your back and glutes against the wall and put your hands behind your head with your feet close together. Lift your right knee and left elbow simultaneously, trying to touch or get them as close together as possible. Perform the same movement with your left knee and right elbow. Alternate as quickly as possible between right and left sides while trying not to lift your back off the wall nor arch your back too much. Inhale with your feet on the floor and exhale as you bring your knee toward your elbow.

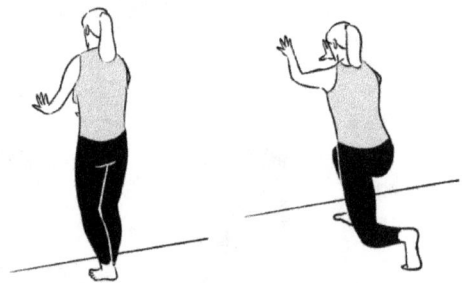

Reverse Lunge
Works: Glutes, Quads, Hip Flexors
Benefits: Balance, Strength & Mobility

Stand facing the wall, an arm's length away, with your feet a few inches apart. Place your hands firmly against the wall, bend your right knee as you step backward with your left leg into a lunge. Go as far back as possible without losing your balance, making sure that only the toes of the left leg touch the floor, and the right knee never goes beyond your toes. Return to the starting position, and repeat on the opposite side. Do this five times on each side.

Day 9

Lunge-Twist

Works: Thighs, Glutes, Shoulders, Core
Benefits: Cardio, Strength & Flexibility

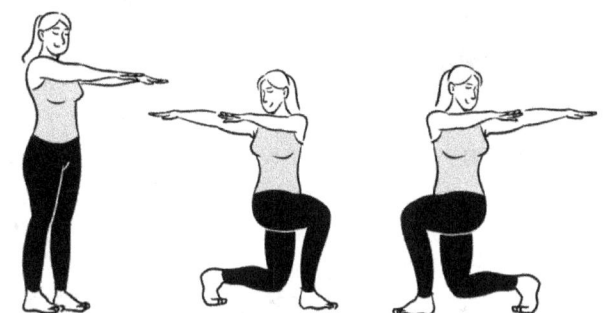

Stand three feet from the wall facing away with your arms extended in front. Bend your left leg backward so that your foot touches the wall. Then, lunge and squat forward with your right leg while twisting your torso to the right. Hold briefly and return to a standing position. Repeat five times then change to the left side.

Thread the Needle

Works: Chest, Shoulders, Triceps
Benefits: Strength & Circulation

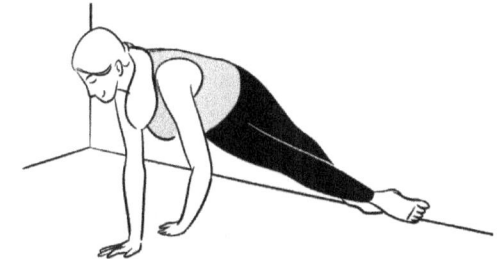

Start on your belly in the push-up position. Place your feet in the crevice between the wall and floor with your left toes touching your right heel. Lift your left arm to the ceiling and then rotate your torso to bring your left arm slowly back down between your chest and the floor. Repeat five times then switch sides.

Child's Pose

Works: Shoulders, Back, Legs
Benefits: Strength, Flexibility & Circulation

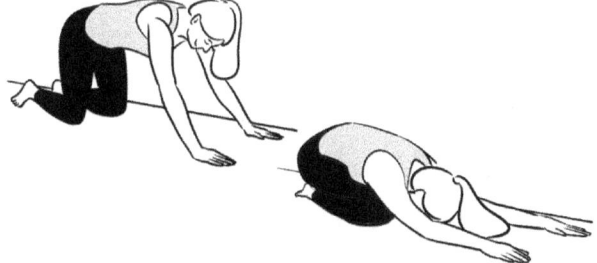

Start on your hands and knees with your arms stretched out slightly in front of you. Keeping your palms on the floor, slowly fold back by bending your knees and folding your upper body so that you are almost sitting on your legs. Hold and look up to stretch the neck. Return to your starting position and repeat.

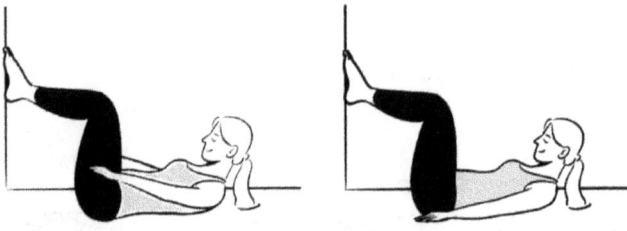

Hundred
Works: Abs, Hips, Core
Benefits: Cardio, Circulation, Strength & Energy

Lie on your back with your knees bent and your feet flat on the wall. Your shins should be in line with the floor and your thighs should be pointing up. Lift your neck and shoulders off the mat to contract your abs and pump your arms by lifting them about a foot up and then back to the mat. Repeat quickly with a goal of 100 total pumps.

This marks the end of "Day 9" exercises.

Day 10

By now, you should be starting to feel stronger and more confident in your moves. Let's start with some warm- ups!

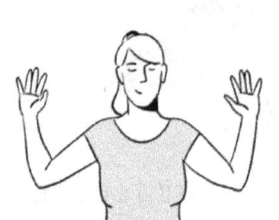 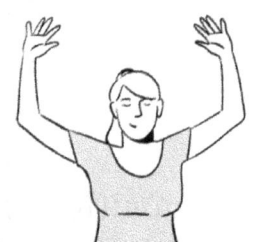

Wall Angels
Works: Upper Back, Scapula, Neck & Shoulders
Benefits: Flexibility & Strength

Start standing with your back against the wall and your feet six inches away. Bend your arms 90 degrees while keeping the backs of your arms and hands flat against the wall. Slowly raise your arms up above your head as far as possible. Use your abs to press your back against the wall. Hold for three seconds at the top and bring back down to the starting position. Repeat five times.

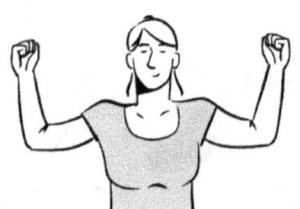 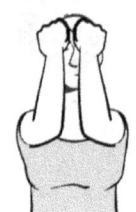

Cactus Arms
Works: Upper Back, Scapula, Neck & Shoulders
Benefits: Flexibility & Strength

Start standing with you rback and the back of your hands and forearms touching the wall. With arms still bent, move them forward so that your palms and forearms come together in front of you. Hold for three seconds. With elbows still bent, move your arms back so your forearms and outer hands tap the wall. Repeat this motion 15-20 times in rapid succession.

Day 10 Main Exercises

Arms Overhead

Works: Chest, Shoulders, Upper Back
Benefits: Strength & Flexibility

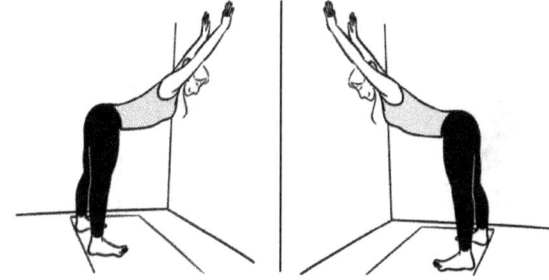

Stand facing the wall, an arm's length away. Raise your arms over your head and place your palms flat against the wall. Keeping your arms straight, lean forward and press your chest towards the wall until you feel a stretch in your upper chest. Hold the stretch for 20-30 seconds, then relax and repeat. For a deeper stretch, put your palms together as you raise your arms and lean forward.

Kneeling Archer

Works: Thoracic spine, Rhomboids, Trapezius
Benefits: Stability, Flexibility, Strength

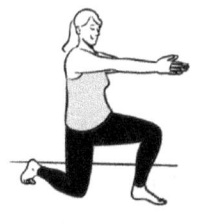 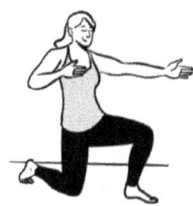 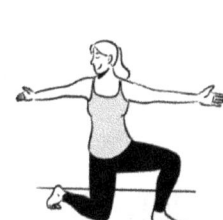 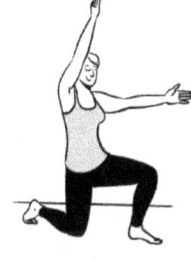 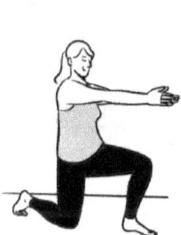

Start by kneeling down on your right knee and your right leg bent so your foot is flat on the floor. Extend your arms in front of you with your palms together. Keep your left arm still as you pull your right arm straight back and rotate your torso while extending your right arm behind you and, in a circular motion, raise your right arm over your head and down in front of you to join the other palm. Repeat three times before switching sides.

Tabletop Reach

Works: Shoulders, Hips, Glutes, Core
Benefits: Cardio, Strength, Flexibility

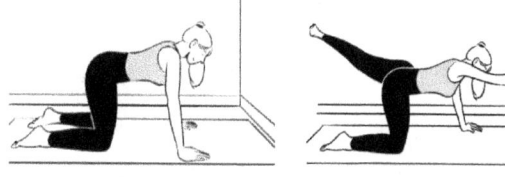

Start in the tabletop position (on hands and knees) facing the wall about an arm's length away. Extend your left leg straight back with toes pointed straight as you simultaneously reach out to the wall with your right hand. Return to neutral position and then extend your right leg out as you touch the wall with your left hand. Do this in rapid, but smooth succession 5-10 times alternating sides each time.

Day 10

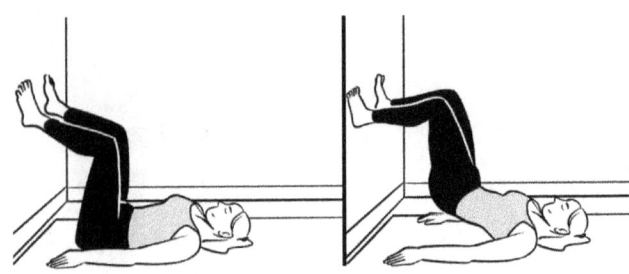

Wall Shoulder Bridge
Works: Core, Glutes, Lower Body
Benefits: Cardio, Strength, Flexibility

The Shoulder bridge is a foundational exercise, perfect for strengthening the core and lower body. Lie on your back with knees bent and your feet on the wall. Flex your glutes and lift your hips in the air and hold for three seconds. Return to starting position and repeat. Depending on your strength level, repeat five to 10 times.

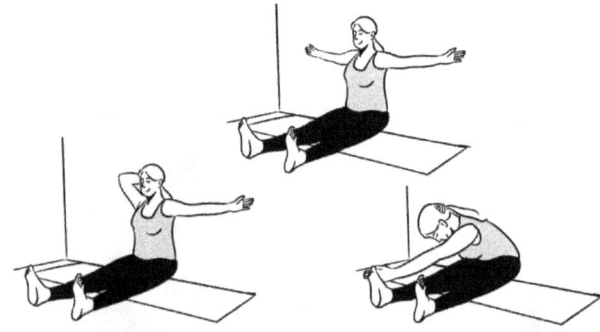

Half Windmill Sit
Works: Core, Obliques, Hips, Thighs
Benefits: Flexibility, Balance, Posture, Coordination

Sit on the floor with your back to the wall and your arms straight out like an airplane. Bend your right elbow to place your right hand on the back of your head. Swing your left arm around to the outside of your RIGHT knee and keeping your back straight, bend to put the back of your left hand on the outside of your right pinky toe. Hold for five seconds then back to neutral position. Repeat on the opposite side.

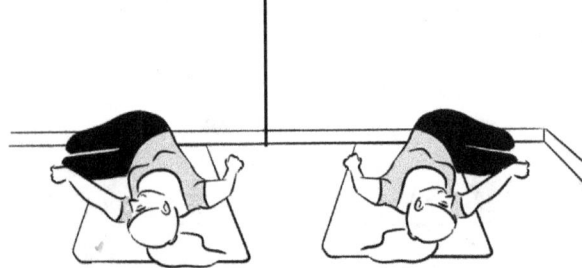

Knee Roll/ Windshield Wiper
Works: Hips, Back, Glutes, Abs
Benefits: Cardio, Strength, Mobility

Start on your back with your arms to your side, knees bent and your feet flat on the wall for spacing. Bring your knees toward your chest slightly and roll your legs to the left until they touch the floor. Hold momentarily and then roll them back to the right until they touch the floor on the right. That's one. Repeat five to ten times. For a more difficult exercise, perform with your legs almost straight.

Day 10

Wall Bicycle
Works: Back, Abs, Hip Flexors, Spine
Benefits: Cardio and Flexibility

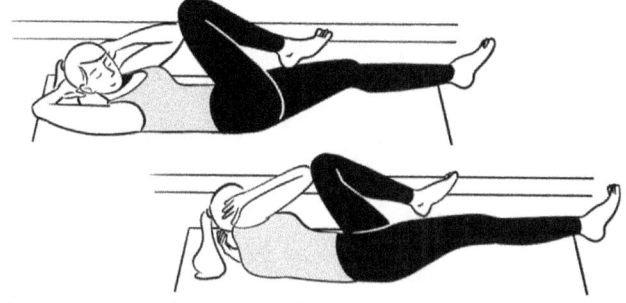

Start on your back with your feet on the wall and your hands behind your head. To start, bring your right knee up as you bend your left elbow down to touch it. Then cross to the opposite side by bringing your left knee up as you bend to touch your right elbow to meet it. That's one. Aim for ten to fifteen repetitions.

Wall Hip Slides
Works: Glutes, Hips
Benefits: Flexibility & Stability

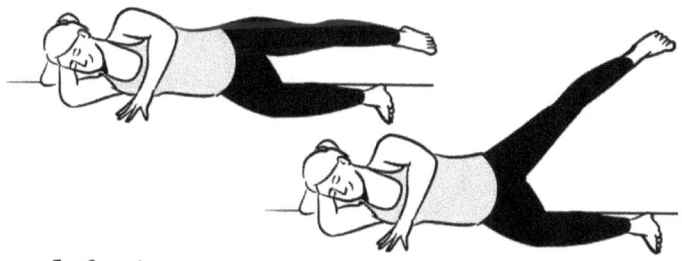

Lie on your side parallel to and facing away from the wall. Both knees should be straight and your top heel should be on the wall. If you want, put a towel between your heel and the wall for smoother movement. Raise your top leg along the wall as high as you can, keeping your heel pressed against the wall. Hold for two seconds then lower. Do this five times then repeat for the opposite side and leg.

Butterfly
Works: Hamstring, Quads, Groin
Benefits: Flexibility, Mobility, Warm-up

Lay on your back and swing your legs up so that your hips and legs are against the wall. Bend your elbows and let your arms rest above your head on the mat. Keeping your feet on the wall, bend your knees in toward your chest while lowering your heels as low as you can and putting the soles of your feet together. Stay in this position while concentrating on breathing for two to three minutes.

To end the Day 10 session, let's do some stretching and breathing.

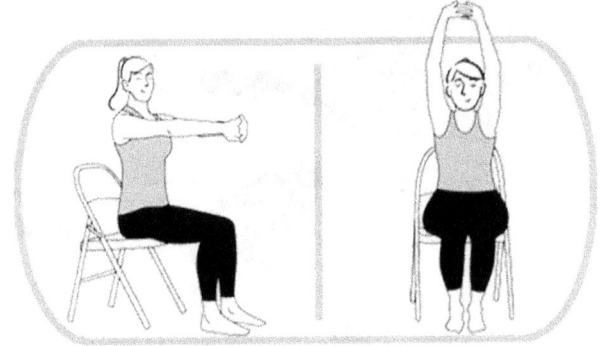

The Scoop
Works: Shoulders, Chest, Spine, Core, Upper Back
Benefits: Flexibility & Breathing

This can be done standing or sitting. With your arms straight down (in your lap if sitting), interlock your fingers with your palms facing up. Inhale as you bring your interlocked palms towards your chin. Turn your interlocked palms outward and exhale slowly as you straighten your elbows until your arms are fully extended. Keep the motion going as you raise your interlocked hands above your head with your palms towards the ceiling. Release your hands and bring them slowly to your sides. Repeat five times.

Belly Breathing
Benefits: Breath Control, Concentration

To start, sit comfortably with your back straight. Place one hand on your chest and the other on your belly. Breathe in deeply through the nose, allowing your belly to expand while keeping your chest still. Hold momentarily and then exhale slowly through your mouth, drawing the belly inward. Breathe in...Breathe out...Pay specific attention to your belly's rise and fall. Once again: Breathe in...Breathe out. Continue for about two minutes.

Box Breathing
Benefits: Stress Relief & Discipline

Also known as "Square Breathing", Box Breathing is particularly effective in reducing stress and managing anxiety. By focusing on slow, deep breaths, it helps counteract the rapid, shallow breathing that often accompanies anxiety. This technique activates the parasympathetic nervous system, signaling the brain to relax and reducing levels of stress hormones like cortisol. Inhale through the nose slowly while counting to four in your head. Hold that breath for a count of four. Exhale through the mouth for a count of four. Hold that breath out for another count of four. Complete 5-10 cycles.

You've made it through Day 10. See you tomorrow!

Day 11-Warm-Ups

As we start today's routines, remember to go at your own pace and intensity. If it's the first time seeing a pose, take some extra time to get the movement right. Now, let's jump into day 11.

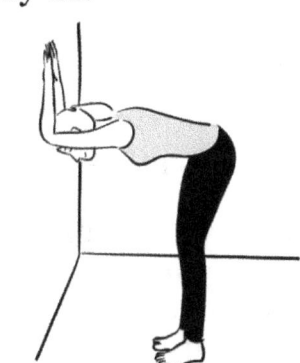

Standing Wall Stretch
Works: Shoulders, Chest, Back
Benefits: Strength & Flexibility

Stand about half an arm's length away and facing the wall. Keeping your legs straight, bend at the hips, put your elbows and forearms on the wall as you breathe in and out. Hold for 10-20 seconds.

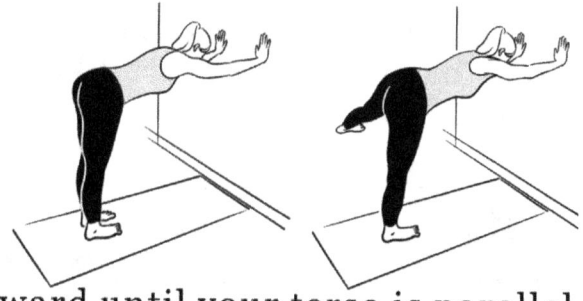

Fwd Bend/Side Leg Lift
Works: Hips, Groin
Benefits: Balance & Cardio

Stand facing the wall and bend forward until your torso is parallel to the floor, your arms straight, and your palms flat against the wall. Lift your left leg out to the side until it's parallel to the floor (or as high as you can), keeping your hips level. Do 10 repetitions and repeat with the right leg. You can also alternate between legs.

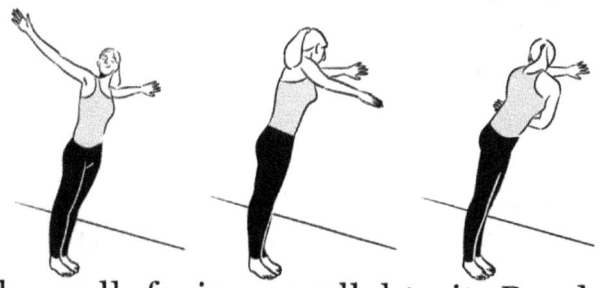

Reach-Twist-Wrap
Works: Chest, Arms and Spine
Benefits: Cardio, Strength, Mobility

Stand an arm's length away from the wall, facing parallel to it. Bend your left arm and put your forearm against the wall. The side of your body should be leaning towards the wall, but straight. Extend right arm out and slightly up behind you and hold briefly. Twist your body to the left while bringing right arm down and under the left arm while keeping it extended and away from the body to "wrap" your body. Inhale as you reach and exhale as you wrap. Complete three to five reps on each side.

Day 11-Main Exercises

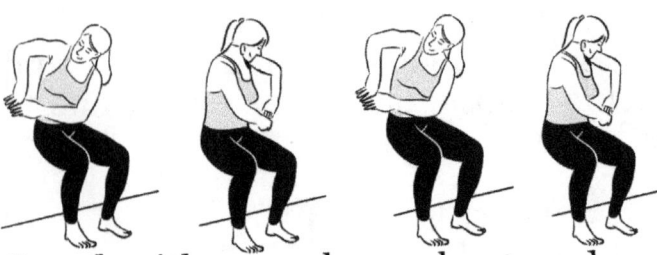

Russian Twist
Works: Abs, Obliques, Spine
Benefits: Cardio, Strength

Stand with your knees bent and your back against the wall in a simi-squat position. Quickly twist your torso to the left while reaching your right arm across your body to touch the wall on your left with your right hand. Twist your torso back to the right while reaching your left arm across your body to touch the wall on your right with your left hand. Quickly repeat this side-to-side motion for 15 to 20 sets of twists. Pause for 10 seconds and repeat.

Bear Sequence

Works: Arms, Shoulders, Hips, Calves, Core   **Benefits:** Balance, Strength, Coordination

These next exercises should flow one to the other. They all use the same basic stance. Start like a bear on all fours with your back straight. This is the "basic position".

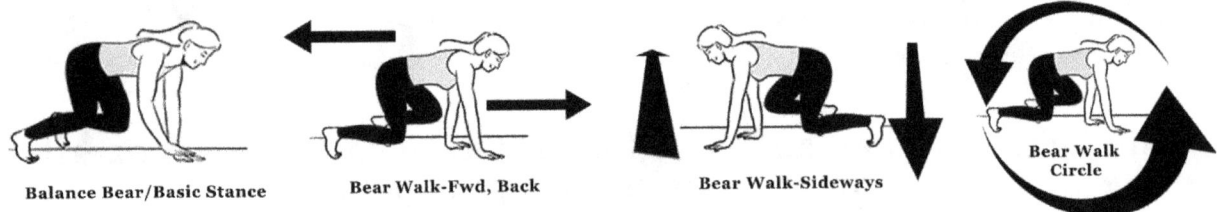

Balance Bear: From the basic position, lift your right hand and your left foot off the floor an inch or two, then replace. Repeat with other side: lift your left hand and your right foot off the floor an inch or two then replace. That's one repetition. Do a total of five to ten reps.

Bear Walk Forward & Backwards: From the basic position, slowly walk across the floor in the balance bear stance then walk backwards back to your starting position. Repeat two times.

Bear Walk-Sideways: From the basic position, walk sideways across the floor in the balance bear stance then sideways back to your starting position. Repeat two times.

Bear Walk-Circle: From the basic position, walk in a wide circle, first clockwise then counter-clockwise. Repeat two times.

Day 11

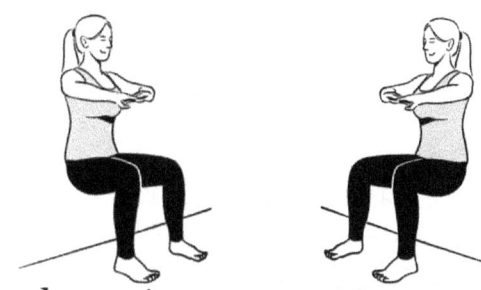

Wall Squat
Works: Quads, Glutes, Hamstrings, Thighs, Hip flexors, Core
Benefits: Strength & Mobility

Stand straight and upright with your hands against your sides and your back against the wall. Walk your feet out in front slightly, then slide down into a squat by bending your knees until thighs are parallel with the floor. Hold momentarily and then push back up. Repeat for 5-10 repetitions. Can also be done with your arms out.

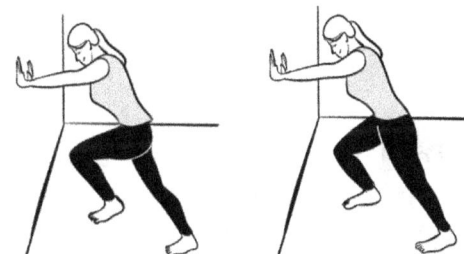

Standing Wall March
Works: Hips, Groin, Quads, Hamstrings
Benefits: Mobility, Balance, Strength

To start, face the wall about one and a half arm's lengths away. Bend your right leg and lift your knee up quickly and bring back down as you switch to the opposite leg and do the same motion. The faster you switch, the more "cardio" the exercise is. One "set" is 10-15 back-and-forth "march" motions between legs. Do two or three sets, resting for 30 seconds between sets.

Wall Scissors
Works: Glutes, Abs, Inner Thighs
Benefits: Strength, Mobility

Lay on your back so that your legs are bent and your legs and buttocks are up against the wall. Stretch your arms out from your side like an airplane. Open your legs widely to stretch the inner thigh and hold for two seconds. Bring back to neutral. Repeat 10 times.

This marks the end of "Day 11" exercises.

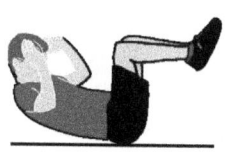 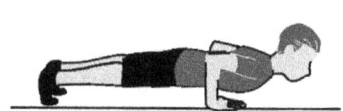 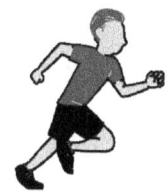 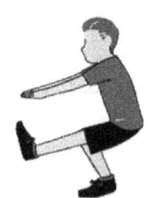

Day 12: Alternate Exercises & Rest

Today you can take a rest from Wall Pilates and enjoy an alternate exercise on your own such as brisk walking, swimming, or biking. You can also do some of the simple stretching and breathing exercises from earlier chapters in the book. We've included a couple of them below.

Belly Breathing

Benefits: Breath Control, Concentration

To start, sit comfortably with your back straight. Place one hand on your chest and the other on your belly. Breathe in deeply through the nose, allowing your belly to expand while keeping your chest still. Hold momentarily and then exhale slowly through your mouth, drawing the belly inward. Breathe in…Breathe out…Pay specific attention to your belly's rise and fall. Once again: Breathe in…Breathe out. Continue for about two minutes.

Box Breathing

Benefits: Stress Relief & Discipline

Also known as "Square Breathing", Box Breathing is particularly effective in reducing stress and managing anxiety. By focusing on slow, deep breaths, it helps counteract the rapid, shallow breathing that often accompanies anxiety. This technique activates the parasympathetic nervous system, signaling the brain to relax and reducing levels of stress hormones like cortisol. Inhale through the nose slowly while counting to four in your head. Hold that breath for a count of four. Exhale through the mouth for a count of four. Hold that breath out for another count of four. Complete 5-10 cycles.

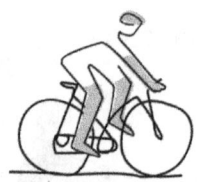 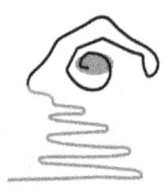 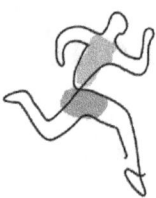 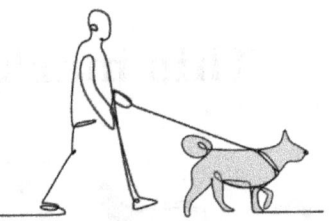

That's it for today's exercises. See you tomorrow for Day 13!

Day 13. Let's start today with "The Scoop"!

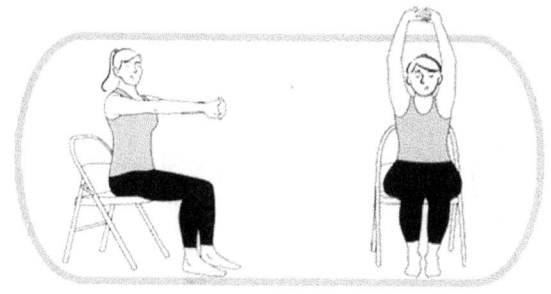

The Scoop
Works: Shoulders, Chest, Spine, Core, Upper Back
Benefits: Flexibility & Breathing

With your arms straight down (in your lap if sitting), interlock your fingers with your palms facing up. Inhale as you bring your interlocked palms towards your chin. Turn your interlocked palms outward and exhale slowly as you straighten your elbows until your arms are fully extended. Keep the motion going as you raise your interlocked hands above your head with your palms towards the ceiling. Release your hands and bring them slowly to your sides. Repeat five times.

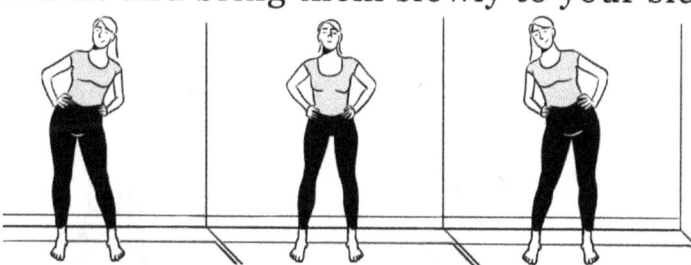

Hip Circles
Works: Hips
Benefits: Flexibility, Mobility, Balance & Strength

Stand facing the wall, with your feet spread shoulder-width apart and about two feet away from the wall. Put your hands on your hips and pull your stomach in so that you engage your core muscle. Bend to the side slightly as you and rotate your hips clockwise 10 times at a medium speed. Repeat in the opposite direction. Gradually increase the size of the circles as you become more flexible and comfortable with the exercise. Benefits the hips for Flexibility, mobility and strength.

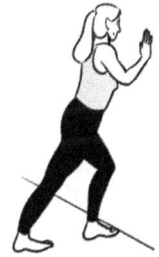 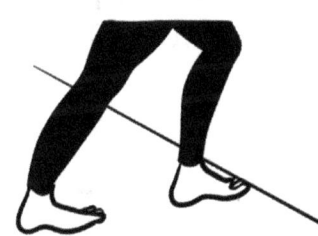

Calf Stretch
Works: Calf Muscles
Benefits: Balance & Mobility

Stand facing the wall about 1 1/2 arms lengths away, feet shoulder length apart. Lean forward to the wall, bend your left knee as you slide the right foot back, keeping your right foot flat on the floor until you feel the stretch in your right calf. Hold for 10 seconds then point your right toe outward continuing the stretch for 10 more seconds. Next, point your right toe inward to stretch for another 10 seconds. Return to neutral position and repeat with the opposite leg and calf.

Day 13

Fwd Bend/Side Leg Lift
Works: Hips, Groin
Benefits: Balance & Cardio

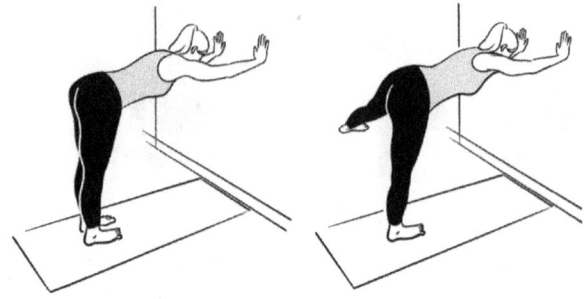

Stand facing the wall and bend forward until your torso is parallel to the floor, your arms straight, and your palms flat against the wall. Lift your left leg out to the side until it's parallel to the floor (or as high as you can), keeping your hips level. Do 10 repetitions and repeat with the right leg. You can also alternate between legs.

Wall-Facing Lunge
Works: Quads, Hamstrings, Glutes
Benefits: Balance, Cardio, Strength

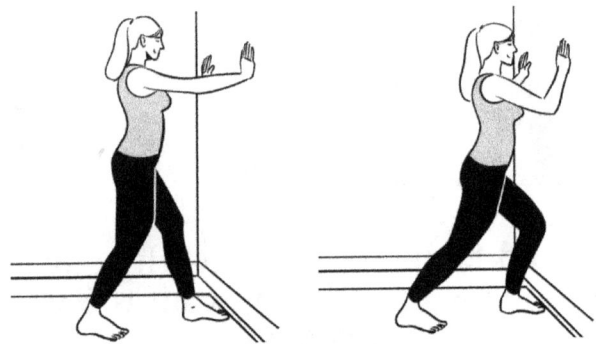

Put your palms on the wall in front of you. Step your left foot forward until your toes nearly touch the wall and move your right foot backwards. Inhale and bend both knees as you bring the left knee close to the wall and your forearms near the wall. The movement should be slow and fluid. Hold for five seconds and repeat with the opposite leg and side. That's one repetition. Do 10 reps.

Sit-Stretch
Works: Back, Shoulders, Waist
Benefits: Flexibility & Mobility

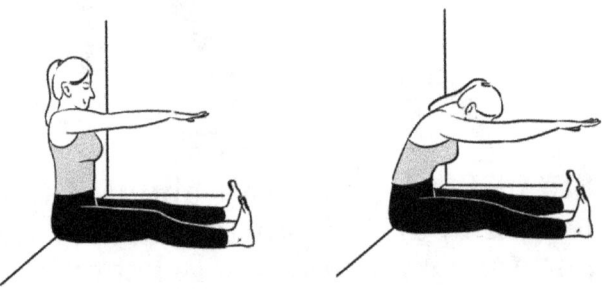

Sit on the floor with your back touching the wall and your arms straight out in front of you. Slowly bend forward, bending at the waist with your head pointed so you are looking at the floor. Go as far as is comfortable and hold for 15-30 seconds. Release and repeat, this time going farther than the first and holding for 30 seconds.

Day 13

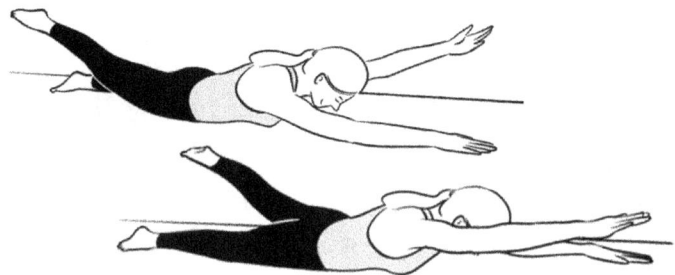

Swimmer's Reach
Works: Abs, Back, Shoulders
Benefits: Flexibility, Mobility

Laying face-down on a mat parallel to the wall, stretch your legs behind you and your arms above your head with palms on the mat. Your head can be up or resting on the mat. Breathe in and raise your locked right arm and left leg straight up at the same time while keeping them parallel to the floor. Hold momentarily and breathe out as you return them to the mat. Repeat with the left arm and right leg. Repeat five times on each side, alternating sides each time. Try and stretch your legs out and reach your arms as much as possible as you perform the movements.

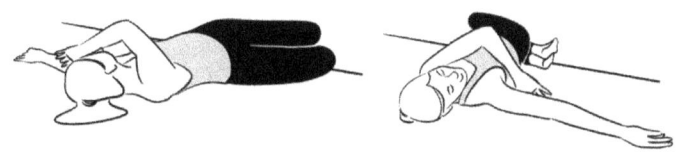

Torso Twist on Mat
Works: Spine, Shoulders, Back
Benefits: Flexibility, Mobility

Lie on your back with your feet touching the wall for reference. Bend your legs at the knees slightly and rotate them to the right so your knees touch the mat. At the same time, extend your arms across your torso to the left, trying to touch the mat on the left side. Hold for three-five seconds and repeat on the opposite sides.

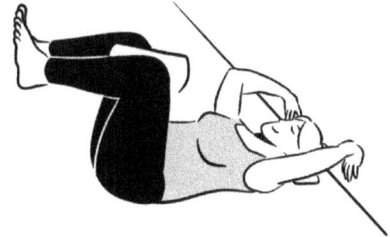

Wall Reverse Crunch
Works: Lower Abs, Quads, Knees
Benefits: Cardio, Strength, Flexibility

Lay on your back with your arms over your head and your palms pressed against the wall. Lift your hips off the ground, bringing your knees toward your chest. Lower your legs back down without touching the floor. Complete three sets of 15 reps. To make it more comfortable, use a small pillow or towel between your knees.

Day 13

Knee Tucks to Chest
Works: Hamstrings, Glutes, Obliques
Benefits: Flexibility, Mobility, Strength

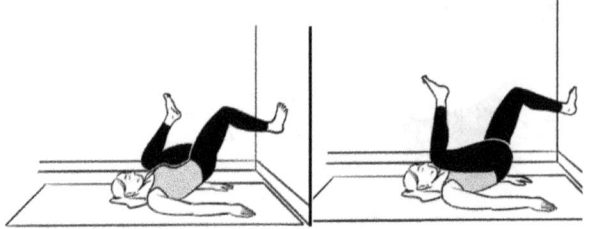

Lay flat on your back and place your knees at a 90° angle against the wall. Extend your arms along your sides. Use your left leg to push towards your chest, lifting your hips (your knee will be towards your chest). Avoid arching your back. Repeat the same movement with your right leg. Inhale as you push and exhale as you bring your foot towards the wall. Repeat ten times.

Multi-Stretch
Works: Spine, Hip Flexors, Hamstrings, Glutes, Obliques
Benefits: Flexibility, Mobility, Strength

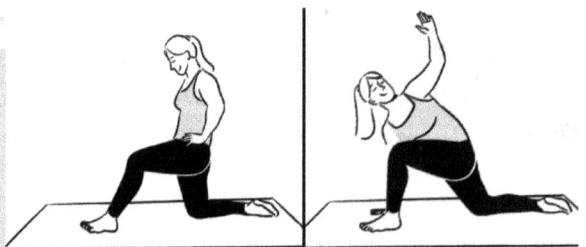

Start on your knees parallel to the wall. Stretch your left leg out in front of you with your leg bent and the foot flat on the floor. Lean forward with your torso to add a stretch to the planted knee's hip flexor. Place right hand on the floor opposite the front foot. Finally, reach your left arm up and rotate towards the ceiling leading with your upper back and shoulders. Hold for 3 seconds then repeat on the opposite side.

The Frog
Works: Knees, Hips, Quads, Groin
Benefits: Balance & Strength

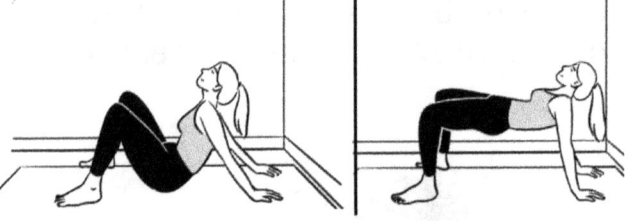

This is an advanced exercise, so start slow and stretch as much as you can without straining. The more you do the move, the farther you'll be able to stretch. Start in a tabletop or "crab walk" position: Your head, stomach and pelvis pointed towards the ceiling with your feet flat on the floor, knees bent and your hands behind you with your palms on the floor. Keep your arms fully extended and not bent. From here, push your buttocks up to straighten your back and stretch your spine as much as possible. Do this three to five times.

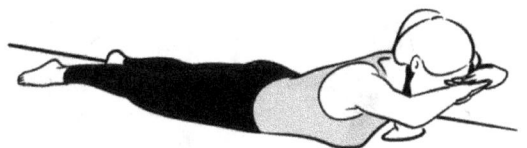

Chest Lift
Works: Back, Abs
Benefits: Posture & Balance

Lay face-down the floor with your elbows bent and your forehead resting on your hands. Breathe in, and as you breathe out, bend at the waist as you lift your arms, head and torso off the mat as far as possible. Hold momentarily and bring back to starting position. Repeat five times.

End of Day 13

Day 14 (Starting with Warm-Ups)

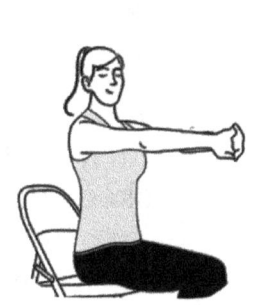 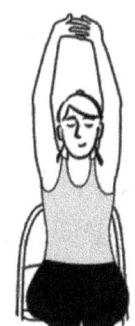

The Scoop
Works: Shoulders, Chest, Spine, Core, Upper Back
Benefits: Flexibility & Breathing

With your arms straight down (in your lap if sitting), interlock your fingers with your palms facing up. Inhale as you bring your interlocked palms towards your chin. Turn your interlocked palms outward and exhale slowly as you straighten your elbows until your arms are fully extended. Keep the motion going as you raise your interlocked hands above your head with your palms towards the ceiling. Release your hands and bring them slowly to your sides. Repeat five times.

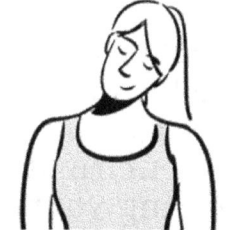 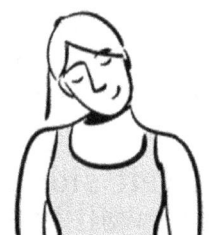

Neck Circles
Works: Neck & Shoulders
Benefits: Warm-Up, Stretch
Tension Release

Stand slightly away from the wall with your arms at your sides. Make five slow, wide circles with your head in each direction. Repeat.

Day 14

Single leg Circles
Works: Quads, Hamstrings, Glutes, Groin
Benefits: Strength, Cardio & Balance

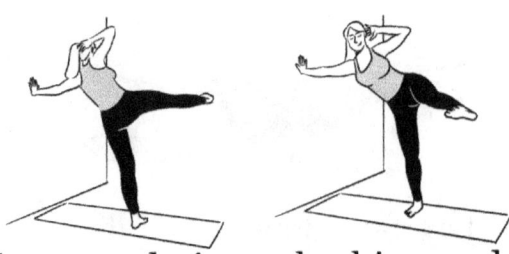

Standing next to the wall, bend slightly towards it at the hips and place your left hand on the wall. Bend your right elbow and put your right hand on the back of your head. Keeping your left leg and back straight, make a wide sweeping circle that goes in front, beside and behind you as much as possible. Do five circles in each direction then switch legs. Do a total of two on each side.

Flamingo
Works: Glutes, Hips, Core, Abs
Benefits: Strength, Posture & Balance

Stand with your back to the wall, with your feet two feet away. Spread your arms like an airplane, with the backs of your arms touching the wall and your palms facing out. Keeping your elbows locked, bring your arms straight out in front of you so that your thumbs are up and your palms are facing each other and nearly touching. Hold briefly and return. That's one. Repeat at a medium speed 15 times.

Lunge Twist
Works: Thighs, Glutes, Shoulders, Core
Benefits: Cardio, Strength, Flexibility

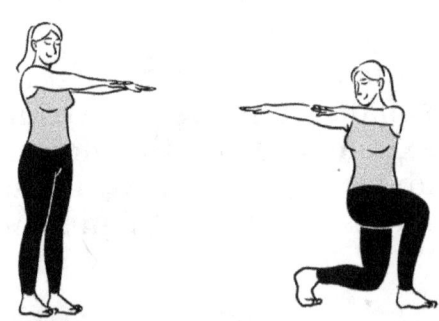

Stand three feet from the wall facing away with your arms extended in front. Bend your left leg backward so that your foot touches the wall. Then, lunge and squat forward with your right leg while twisting your torso to the right. Hold briefly and return to a standing position. Repeat five times then change to the left side. Bend your right leg backward so that your foot touches the wall while bending your left leg out as you lunge forward and twist your torso to the left. Hold briefly and return to a standing position.

Day 14

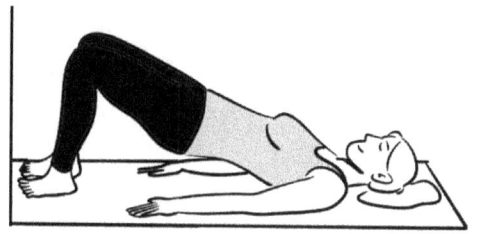

Floor Glute Bridge
Works: Knees, Hips, Quads, Groin & Glutes
Benefits: Strength & Balance

Lie on your back with your feet flat on the floor, toes touching the wall, and your knees bent at a 90-degree angle. Make sure your back is flat against the mat. Lift your hips towards the ceiling and squeeze your glutes. Hold for five seconds, and then relax. Repeat ten times.

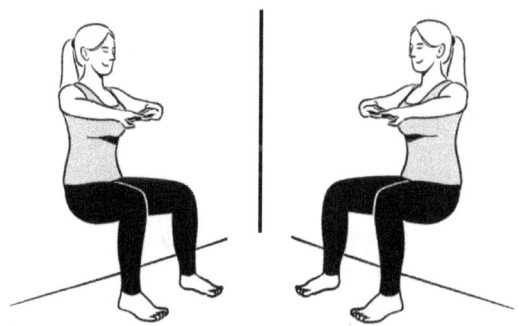

Wall Sit
Works: Quadriceps, Hams, Glutes,
Benefits: Knee Stability and Mobility

Stand with your back against the wall with your feet shoulder-width apart. walk your feet out slightly so that your back is leaning against the wall slightly. Slowly lower your body down the wall, keeping your feet flat on the floor. Stop when your thighs are parallel to the floor. If you can't see your toes, your feet are too far in towards the wall. Stay in this parallel squat position for 30 seconds.

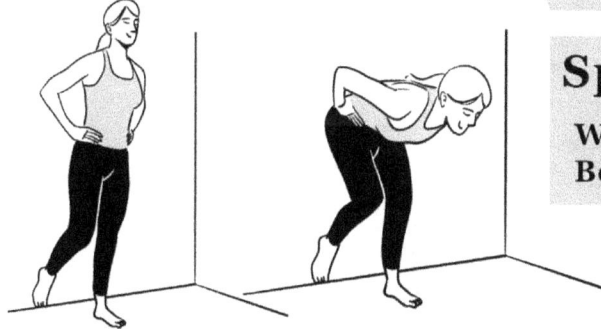

Split Stance Deadlift
Works: Glutes, Hamstring, Quads, Core
Benefits: Strength, balance, Coordination

Stand with your back to the wall, both feet about a foot away. Place your right heel behind you on the wall with toes on the floor. With both knees slightly bent, bend at your hips keeping your back flat. Keep your front knee over your front ankle and tighten your core. Once your upper body is about parallel to floor, use your right foot to stand up, extending your hips. Do 8-10 reps. then switch sides.

Day 14

Bear Sequence

Works: Arms, Shoulders, Hips, Calves, Core   **Benefits:** Balance, Strength, Coordination

These next exercises should flow one to the other. They all use the same basic stance. Start like a bear on all fours with your back straight. This is the "basic position".

Balance Bear: From the basic position, lift your right hand and your left foot off the floor an inch or two, then replace. Repeat with other side: lift your left hand and your right foot off the floor an inch or two then replace. That's one repetition. Do a total of five to ten reps.

Bear Walk Forward & Backwards: From the basic position, slowly walk across the floor in the balance bear stance then walk backwards back to your starting position. Repeat two times.

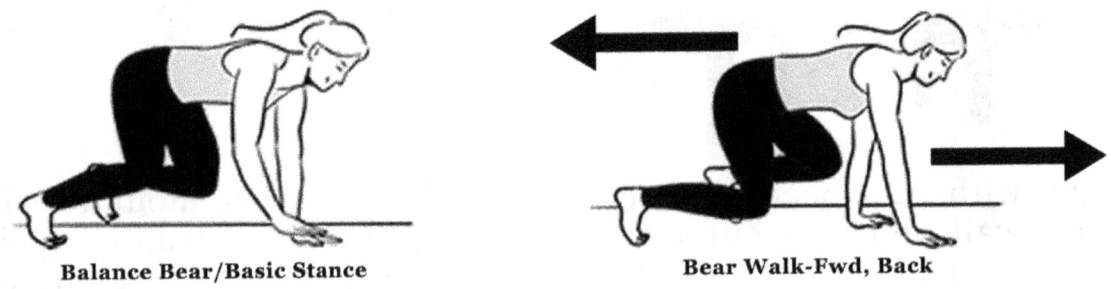

Balance Bear/Basic Stance   Bear Walk-Fwd, Back

Bear Walk-Sideways: From the basic position, walk sideways across the floor in the balance bear stance then sideways back to your starting position. Repeat two times.

Bear Walk-Circle: From the basic position, walk in a wide circle, first clockwise then counter-clockwise. Repeat two times.

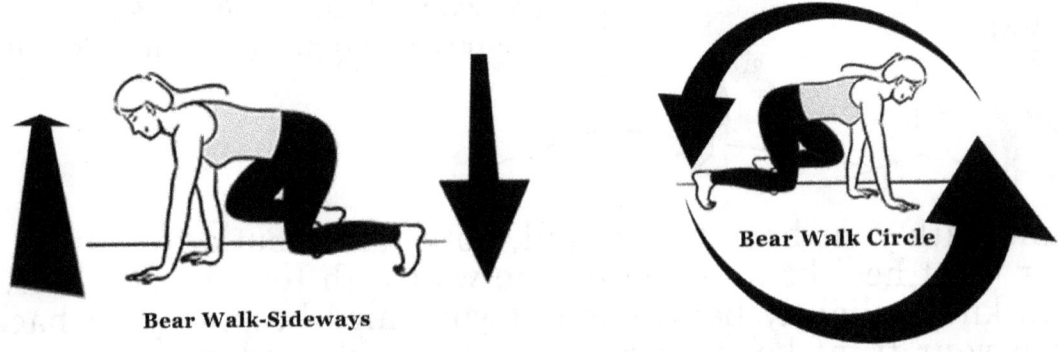

Bear Walk-Sideways   Bear Walk Circle

Congratulations! You've made it halfway through the 28-Day Success Plan. See you in the next chapter for Part 2.

Chapter 7
28-Day Success Plan-Part 2
Days 15-28

You're at the halfway point! Some of these exercises should be second nature by now, but if you need a refresher, remember to refer to the videos to jog your memory. You can access these along with the free illustration chart in Chapter 13.

As you start the second half of the 28-Day Plan, you might notice that the routines are getting longer and progressively more difficult. Changing it up, adding rest days, or modifying the routines to fit your current level is ok. Remember that form is more important than intensity and number of repetitions. With that in mind, turn the page and let's start Day 15 with warm-ups and stretches.

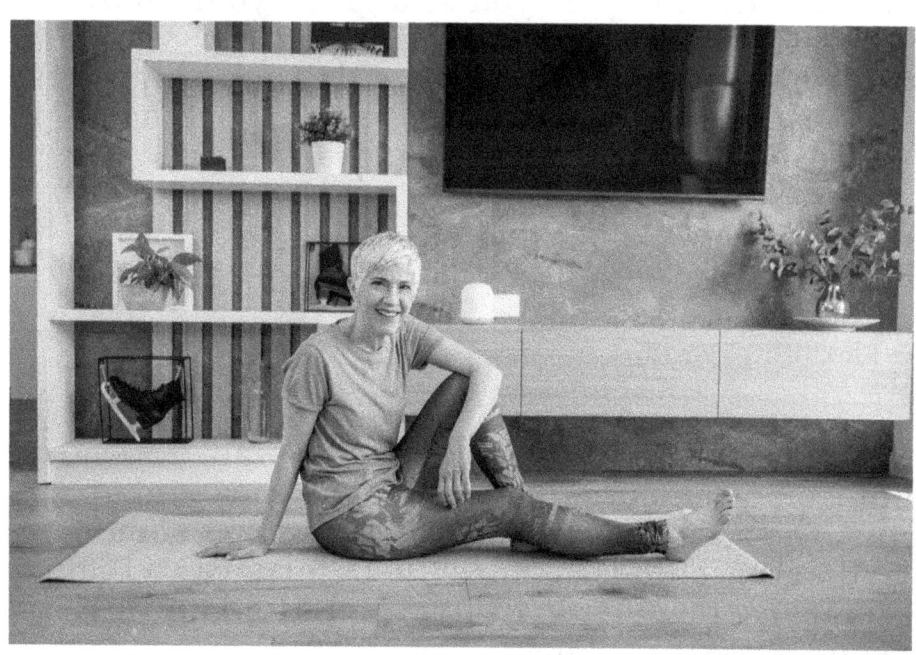

Day 15. Starting with warm-ups

Tricep/Scapula Stretch
Works: Shoulders, Chest, Spine, Upper Back
Benefits: Warm-up & Flexibility

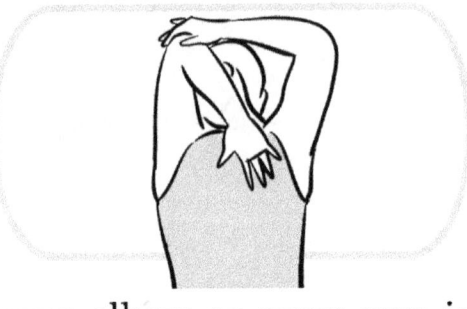

Raise your left arm overhead and bend your elbow so your arm is behind your head and you hand on your upper back. Use your right arm to pull the elbow closer to your head and push down slightly. Hold the stretch for 30 seconds. Repeat with the opposite arm and two times each side.

The Scoop
Works: Shoulders, Chest, Spine, Back
Benefits: Posture, Flexibility, Breathing

Begin with your arms straight down (in your lap if sitting), interlock your fingers with your palms facing up. Inhale as you slowly bring your interlocked palms towards your chin. Turn your interlocked palms outward and exhale slowly as you straighten your elbows until your arms are fully extended. Keep the motion going as you raise your interlocked hands above your head with your palms towards the ceiling. Hold momentarily, and then release your hands and bring them slowly to your sides. Repeat five times.

Cactus Arms
Works: Back, Chest, Shoulders
Benefits: Flexibility, Warm-Up

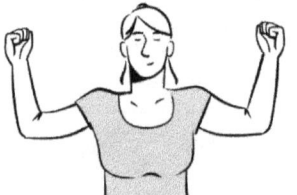 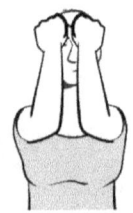

Start with your back and body against the wall. Extend your arms straight out from your sides like an airplane and bend up at the elbow like a cactus. The back of your hands and forearms should be touching the wall. With arms still bent, move them forward so that your palms and forearms come together in front of you. Hold for three second and return to start. Repeat 15 times.

Day 15 Main Exercises

Wall Push-Up

Works: Shoulders, Chest, Back
Benefits: Strength, Posture

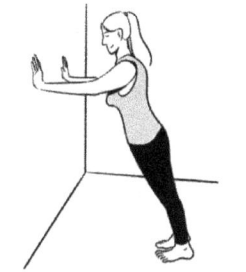
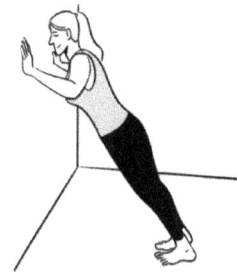

Stand about an arms' length from a wall. Place your palms flat on the wall, slightly wider than shoulder-width apart, with your arms straight, and your fingers pointing upward. Take a small step back, so you are leaning against your hands. Keeping your spine straight, slowly bend your arms until your head touches the wall. Pause. Slowly push yourself away from the wall and back up. That's one. Do this ten to fifteen times.

Side Bend with Leg Lift

Works: Lats, Hips and Groin
Benefits: Flexibility, Mobility, Balance

Stand sideways, an arm's length from the wall, with your right side closest to the wall and feet hip-width apart. Put your right forearm on the wall, extend your left arm overhead, and slide your right hand down the wall as you bend your torso to the right. Hold this position and lift your left leg up and out sideways for ten repetitions. Switch sides and repeat.

Lateral Split Squat

Works: Knees, Hips, Groin
Benefits: Flexibility, Mobility, Balance

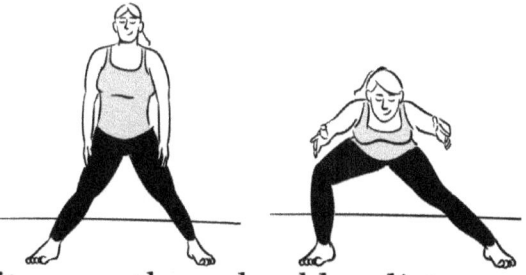

Start by standing with both feet a bit more than shoulder distance apart. Keeping both feet on the floor, lean towards one leg and bend the knee and hip to lower the body. Continue to lower the body until your thigh is parallel to the floor. Press downwards with your foot to push your body back up into neutral position. Repeat with the opposite leg and three to five times each side.

Day 15

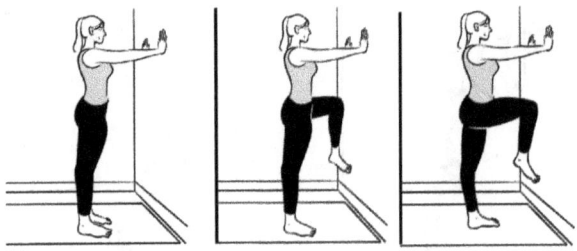

Mountain Climb
Works: Cardio, Core, Abs
Benefits: Strength, Balance, Cardio

Stand an arm's length away with your hands on the wall and your arms fully extended but not bent. To start, bend your leg and lift your right knee towards the wall with your toes and lower leg pointed down. Immediately return to start and repeat with the left leg, while keeping your back straight. The movements should be controlled, but quick. Repeat the back-and-forth motion for 10-15 reps..

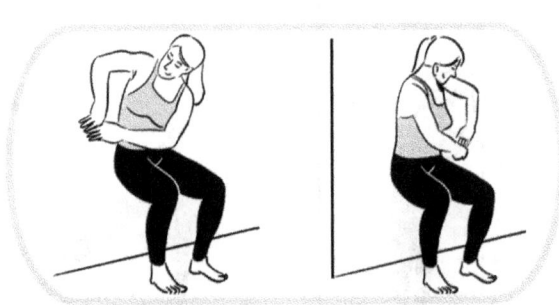

Russian Twists
Works: Abs, Back/Spine, Shoulders
Benefits: Cardio & Strength

Stand with your knees bent and your back against the wall in a simi-squat position. Quickly twist your torso to the left while reaching your right arm across your body to touch the wall on your left with your right hand. Twist your torso back to the right while reaching your left arm across your body to touch the wall on your right with your left hand. Quickly repeat this side-to-side motion for 15 to 20 sets of twists.

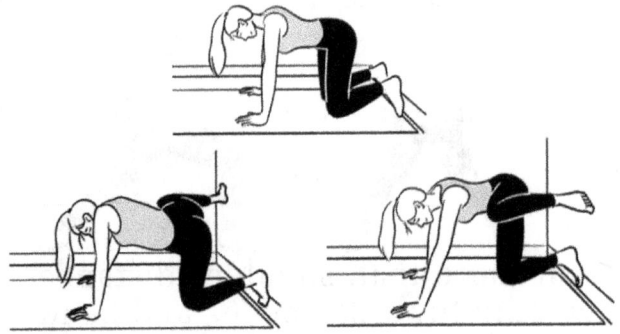

Knee Raises on Mat
Works: Hip Flexors, Obliques
Benefits: Cardio, Balance, Mobility

Start on your hands and knees with your toes an inch from the wall behind you. Keeping your back and arms straight and knee bent, spread your legs apart by lifting your bent right leg out and up towards the ceiling. Hold momentarily and then back to the floor. Do 10 times on each side.

Day 15

Tabletop Reach
Works: Shoulders, Hips, Glutes, Core
Benefits: Cardio, strength, flexibility

Start on your hands and knees facing the wall about an arm's length away. Extend your left leg straight back with toes pointed straight as you simultaneously reach out to the wall with your right hand. Return to neutral position and then extend your right leg out as you touch the wall with your left hand. Do this in rapid, but smooth succession 5-10 times alternating sides each time.

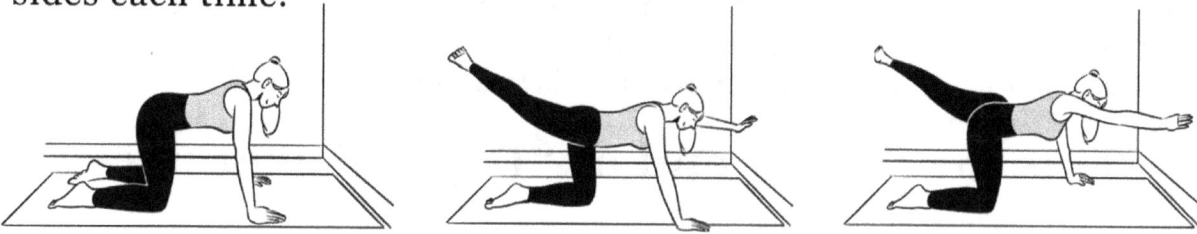

Knee Extension
Works: Abs, Quadriceps
Benefits: Strength, Balance, Flexibility

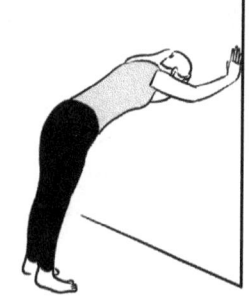
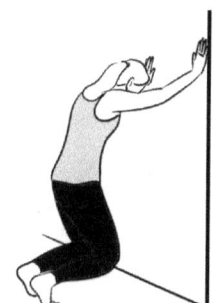

Start by facing the wall about one and a half arm's lengths away. Raise your arms above your head or lean over and place your hands on the wall without bending your knees. Keeping your feet in place, slowly bend at the knees towards the wall and hold momentarily before coming back to the starting position. Do this 5-10 times.

Elevated Glute Bridge
Works: Legs, Shoulders, Glutes, Abs
Benefits: Strength, Mobility, Balance

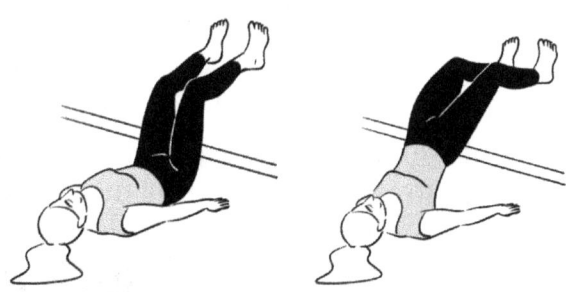

Lie faceup and place your feet flat on a wall about hip-width apart with your knees and hips bent at 90-degree angles and your arms at your sides. Lift your hips until your body makes a straight line from your knees to your shoulders. Squeeze your glutes, then lower back to the floor. Do five to 10 repetitions.

Day 15

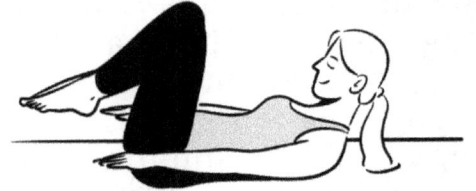

The Hundred
Works: Cardio, Core, Abs
Benefits: Strength, Balance, Cardio

(Intermediate Level) Lie on your back with your knees bent and pointed slightly toward your head and the bottom of your feet parallel to floor. Elevate your arms to a 45-degree angle, in line with your thighs. Then, lift your neck and shoulders off the mat, squeezing your upper abs. Pump your arms as you inhale and exhale slowly. Aim for a total of 100 pumps. Do this two times.

This marks the end of "Day 15" exercises.

Day 16: Alternate Exercises & Rest

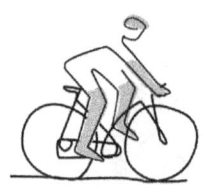 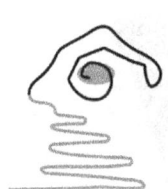 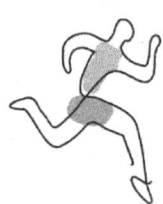 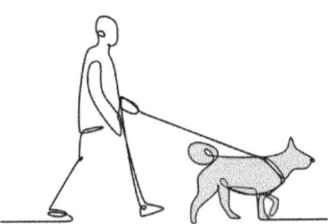

Today you can take a rest from Wall Pilates and enjoy an alternate exercise on your own such as brisk walking, swimming, or biking. You can also do some of the simple stretching and breathing exercises from earlier chapters in the book. We've included instructions for two basic breathing exercises below.

Belly Breathing
Benefits: Breath Control, Concentration

To start, sit comfortably with your back straight. Place one hand on your chest and the other on your belly. Breathe in deeply through the nose, allowing your belly to expand while keeping your chest still. Hold momentarily and then exhale slowly through your mouth. Continue for about two minutes.

Box Breathing
Benefits: Stress Relief & Discipline

Inhale through the nose slowly while counting to four in your head. Hold that breath for a count of four. Exhale through the mouth for a count of four. Hold that breath out for another count of four. Complete 5-10 cycles.

Day 17. We're starting today with some familiar warm-ups.

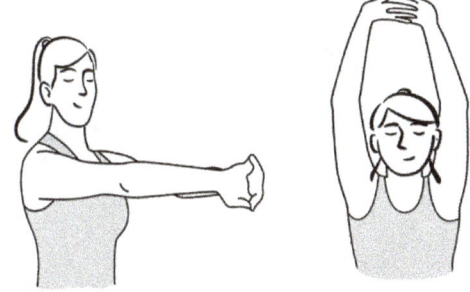

The Scoop
Works: Shoulders, Chest, Spine, Upper Back
Benefits: Posture, Flexibility, Breathing

Interlock your fingers in your lap with your palms facing up and inhale as you bring your interlocked palms towards your chin. Exhale slowly as you straighten your elbows and turn you interlocked palms outward until your arms are fully extended. While continuing to exhale, keep the motion going as you raise your interlocked hands above your head with your palms towards the ceiling. Release your hands, face your palms out and bring them slowly to your sides. Repeat five times.

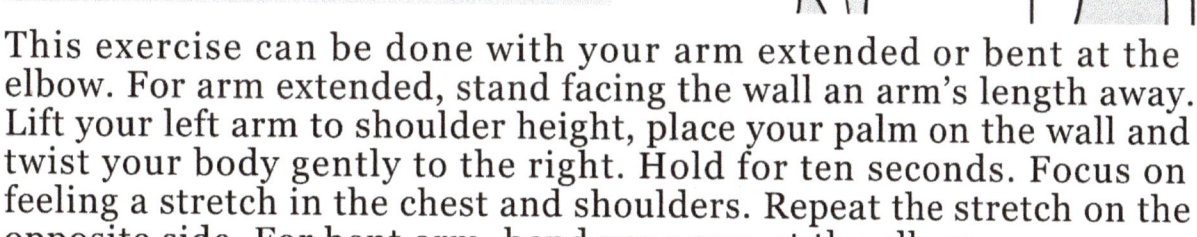

Single Arm Pec Stretch
Works: Back, Chest, Shoulders
Benefits: Flexibility, Warm-Up

This exercise can be done with your arm extended or bent at the elbow. For arm extended, stand facing the wall an arm's length away. Lift your left arm to shoulder height, place your palm on the wall and twist your body gently to the right. Hold for ten seconds. Focus on feeling a stretch in the chest and shoulders. Repeat the stretch on the opposite side. For bent arm, bend your arm at the elbow.

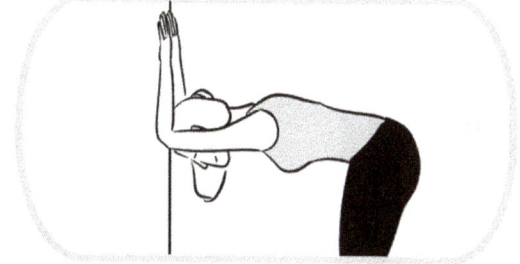

Standing Wall Stretch
Works: Shoulders, Chest, Back
Benefits: Flexibility, Warm-Up

Stand about half an arm's length away and facing the wall. Keeping your legs straight, bend at the hips, put your elbows and forearms on the wall as you breathe out. Hold for 5-10 seconds while breathing in and out slowly and deeply. Repeat five times or as an energizing and stretching routine between other exercises.

Day 17

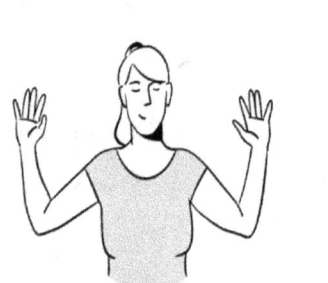 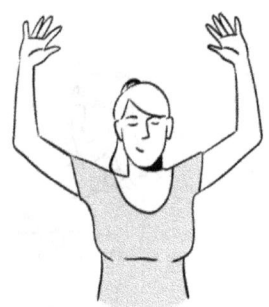

Wall Angels
Works: Back, Chest, Shoulders
Benefits: Flexibility, Warm-Up

Stand with your back to the wall and feet about six inches away. Bend your arms 90 degrees while keeping them as flat against the wall as possible. From that position, keep your back and arms on the wall and slowly raise your arms up as far as possible. Use your abs to press your back against the wall. Hold briefly at the top and bring back down to the starting position. Repeat five to ten times.

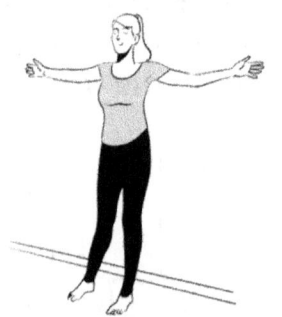 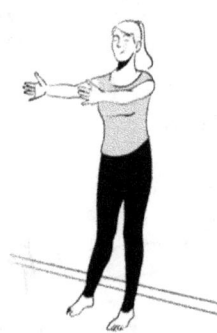

Bird Flap
Works: Scapula, Chest, Shoulders
Benefits: Flexibility, Balance

Stand with you back to the wall, glutes and shoulders touching. Your feet should be about two feet away, your arms straight out like an airplane, with the backs of your arms and hands touching the wall and your palms facing out. Keeping your elbows locked, bring your arms straight out in front of you so that your thumbs are up and your palms are facing each other and nearly touching. Hold momentarily and then return your arms to the wall. That's one. Repeat at a medium speed 15 times then rest for 10 seconds and repeat.

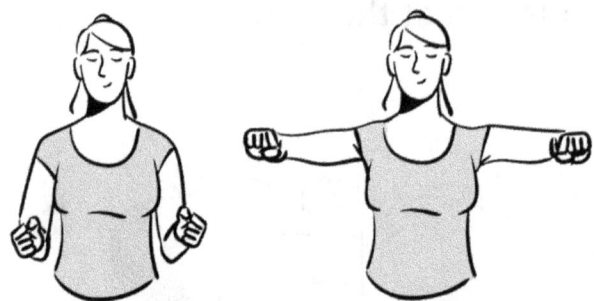

Arm Raises on the Wall
Works: Back and Spine
Benefits: Posture and Mobility

Stand upright, feet shoulder-width apart with your back against the wall so that your head, buttocks, and upper back are firmly pressed against it. Spread your arms like an airplane against the wall and, keeping your upper arms against the wall, bend your elbows so that that your forearms are pointed in front of you. Keep you upper arms against the wall and raise your elbows up toward the ceiling. Repeat 5-10 times.

Day 17

Wall Push-Ups
Works: Chest, Back, Shoulders, Triceps
Benefits: Strength & Circulation

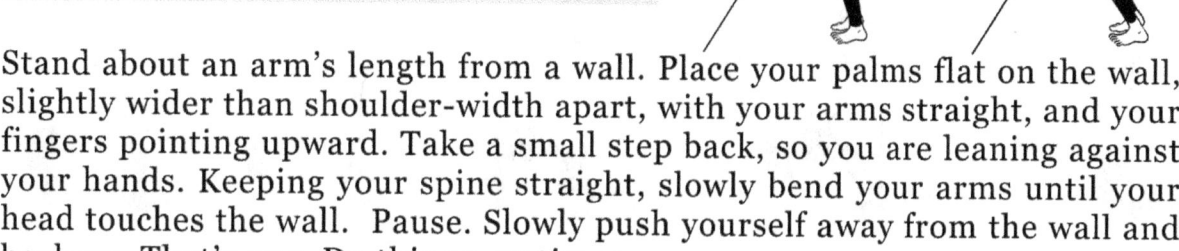

Stand about an arm's length from a wall. Place your palms flat on the wall, slightly wider than shoulder-width apart, with your arms straight, and your fingers pointing upward. Take a small step back, so you are leaning against your hands. Keeping your spine straight, slowly bend your arms until your head touches the wall. Pause. Slowly push yourself away from the wall and back up. That's one. Do this 10-15 times.

Thread the Needle
Works: Chest, Shoulders, Triceps
Benefits: Flexibility, Warm-Up

Start on your belly in the push-up position. Place your feet in the crevice between the wall and floor with your left toes touching your right heel. Lift your left arm to the ceiling and then rotate your torso to bring your left arm slowly back down between your chest and the floor. Repeat five times then switch sides. Place your right foot behind your left with your toes touching your left heel. Lift your right arm to the ceiling and then rotate your torso to bring your arm slowly back down between your chest and the floor. Repeat five times.

Lunge Twist
Works: Legs, Back, Spine, Shoulders
Benefits: Cardio & Strength

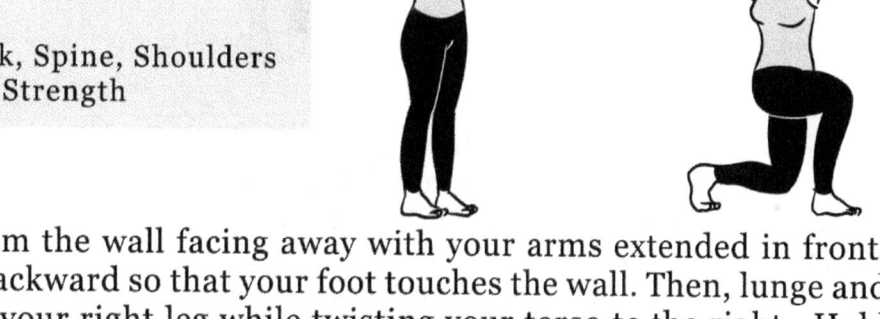

Stand three feet from the wall facing away with your arms extended in front. Bend your left leg backward so that your foot touches the wall. Then, lunge and squat forward with your right leg while twisting your torso to the right. Hold briefly and return to a standing position. Repeat five times then change to the left side. Bend your right leg backward so that your foot touches the wall while bending your left leg out as you lunge forward and twist your torso to the left. Hold briefly and return to a standing position.

Day 17

Kneeling Archer

Works: Thoracic spine, Rhomboids, Trapezius

Benefits: Stability, Flexibility, Strength

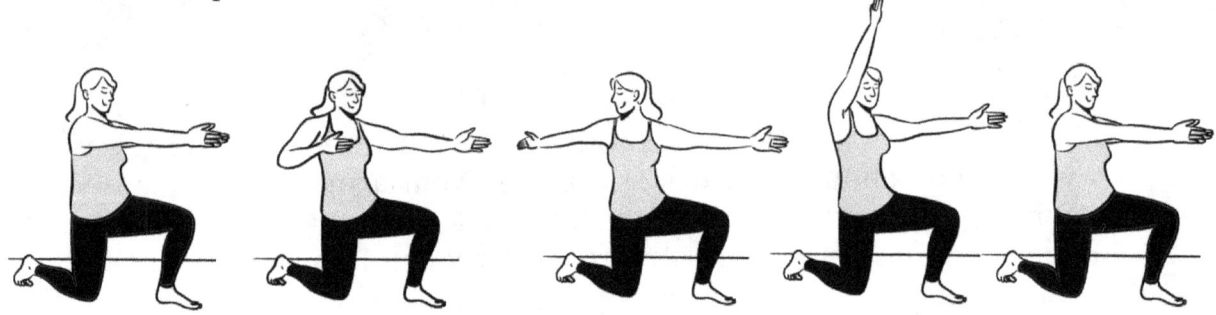

Start by kneeling down on your right knee and your right leg bent so your foot is flat on the floor. Extend your arms in front of you with your palms together. Keep your left arm still as you pull your right arm straight back and rotate your torso while extending your right arm behind you and, in a circular motion, raise your right arm over your head and down in front of you to join the other palm. Repeat three times before switching sides.

Wall Sit, Leg Out

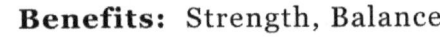

Works: Quads, Hamstrings, Glutes

Benefits: Strength, Balance

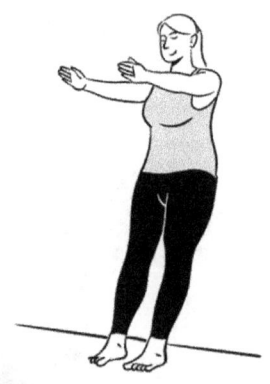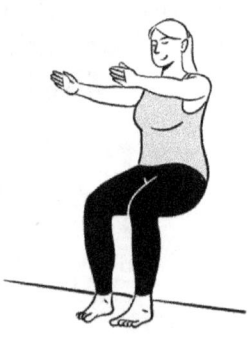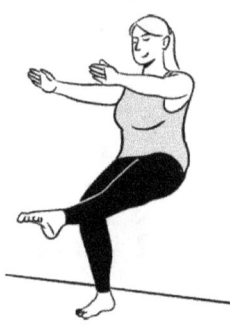

Stand with your back on the wall and your feet shoulder-width apart. Keep your hands at your sides or hold them out in front of you for balance. Bend your knees, lowering your hips deeply so your thighs are parallel with the floor, keeping weight back on your heels. Slowly raise your right leg out so that it is straight with your toes pointed. Hold for 30 seconds. Rise back up and repeat the motion, this time raising the right leg. Relax. Repeat up to three times.

This marks the end of exercises for Day 17. See you tomorrow!

Day 18. Today, we'll focus on the core, but first, a few warm-up stretches.

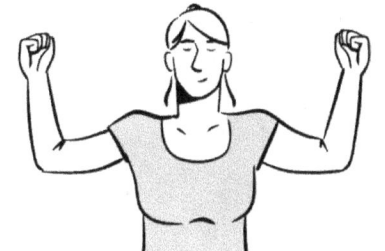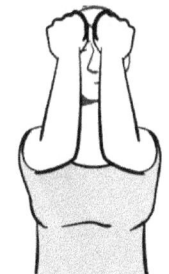

Cactus Arms
Works: Back, Chest, Shoulders
Benefits: Flexibility, Warm-Up

Start with your back and body against the wall. Extend your arms straight out from your sides like an airplane and bend up at the elbow like a cactus. The back of your hands and forearms should be touching the wall. With arms still bent, move them forward so that your palms and forearms come together in front of you. Hold for three second and return to start. Repeat 15 times.

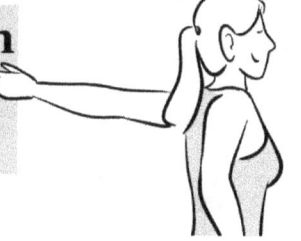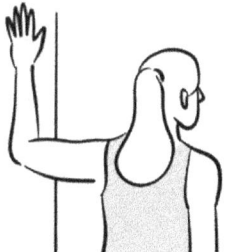

Single Arm Pec Stretch
Works: Back, Chest, Shoulders
Benefits: Flexibility, Warm-Up

This exercise can be done with your arm extended or bent at the elbow. For arm extended, stand facing the wall an arm's length away. Lift your left arm to shoulder height, place your palm on the wall and twist your body gently to the right. Hold for ten seconds. Focus on feeling a stretch in the chest and shoulders. Repeat the stretch on the opposite side. For bent arm, bend your arm at the elbow.

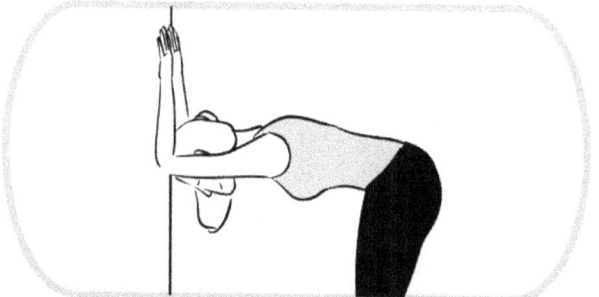

Standing Wall Stretch
Works: Back, Chest, Shoulders
Benefits: Flexibility, Warm-Up

Stand about half an arm's length away and facing the wall. Keeping your legs straight, bend at the hips and put your elbows and forearms on the wall as you breathe out. Hold for 5-10 seconds.

Day 18 Main Exercises

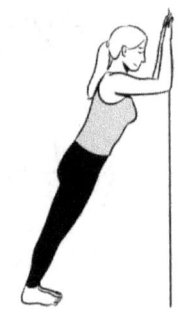

Wall Plank
Works: Triceps, Scapula, Core
Benefits: Warm-Up, Strength

Stand facing the wall about one and a half arm's length away. Lean into the wall, bend your arms and place your forearms and hands on the wall with your palms touching the wall. Hold this position for 30 seconds to two minutes making sure to keep your spine in a straight line. Do not let your hips bend in to the wall!

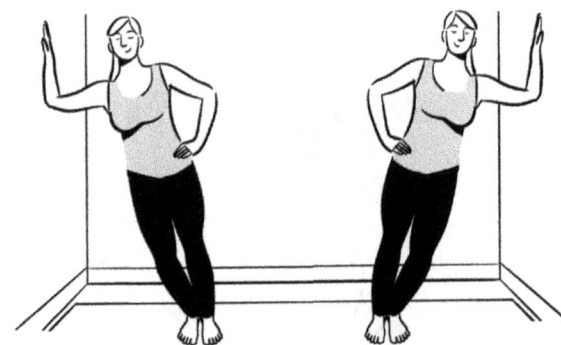

Side Plank
Works: Obliques, Shoulders, Core
Benefits: Warm-Up, Strength

Stand next to the wall about three feet away. Put your right hand on your right hip and bend your left elbow in a 90-degree angle. Keep your body straight, lean sideways and place your left forearm on the wall so it's supporting you on the wall. Hold for 15 to 30 seconds on each side. Do three sets.

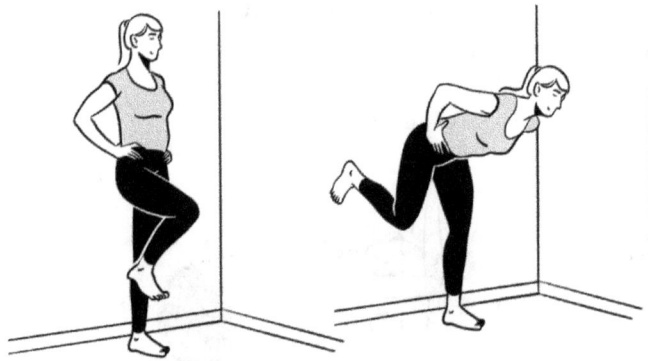

Flamingo
Works: Glutes, Hips, Core, Abs
Benefits: Balance, Coordination, Strength & Mobility

Stand on your left leg with your right leg bent so that your knee is pointed straight out and your right foot is up next to your left knee. Place your hands on your hips to balance, bend forward, extending your right leg back and up to touch the wall behind you. Hold briefly, then return to the start. Do five reps, then switch to having the left up while standing on your right leg.

Day 18

Reach-Twist-Wrap
Works: Chest, Arms, Spine
Benefits: Strength, Fitness

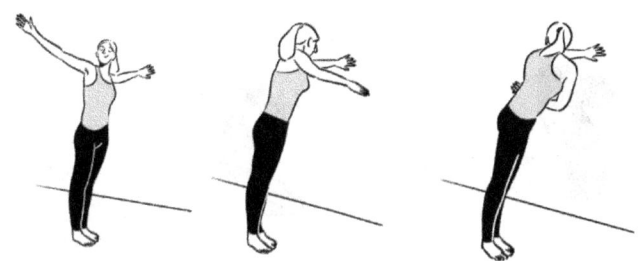

Stand an arm's length away from wall, facing parallel to it. Bend your left arm, lean your body and place your forearm against the wall while keeping your side straight. Reach your right arm out to your side and slightly up and hold briefly as you inhale. Exhale and twist your body to the left while bringing your right arm down and under the left arm while keeping it extended and away from you to "wrap" your body.

Wall Tree (No Chair)
Works: Core, Shoulders, Pelvis
Benefits: Balance, Coordination, Strength, Mobility

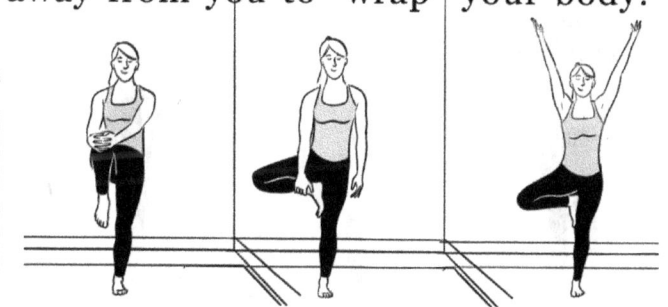

For beginners, use the wall for balance, or use a chair as described below. Once you are comfortable with the exercise, do it away from the wall, but close enough for safety. To start, stand facing away from the wall slightly and bend your right knee, grabbing it with your hands, pausing until you are stable. Then, grab your right foot with your right hand, twisting it slightly so that the inner thigh is looking upward. Bring it up slowly-as high as you can against your left leg with the bottom of your right foot against the side of your left leg. Lock it in if possible then swing your arms up over your head. Hold for 30-60 seconds and then release. Repeat with the left leg.

Wall Tree with Chair
Works: Core, Shoulders, Pelvis
Benefits: Balance, Coordination, Strength, Mobility

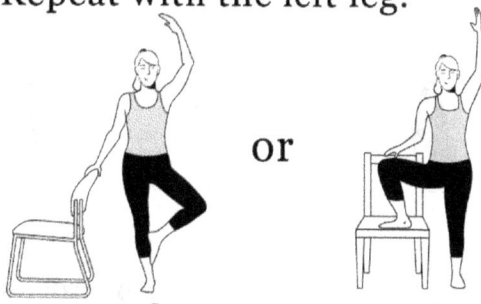

If you need a bit more safety, you can use a chair. Stand beside your chair, holding onto the backrest with your right hand for support. Put your right foot flat on the ground, lift your left foot, and place it against your inner thigh or the calf of your right leg, avoiding the knee area. Bring your right arm up above your head and hold for three breaths. Switch sides and repeat.

Day 18

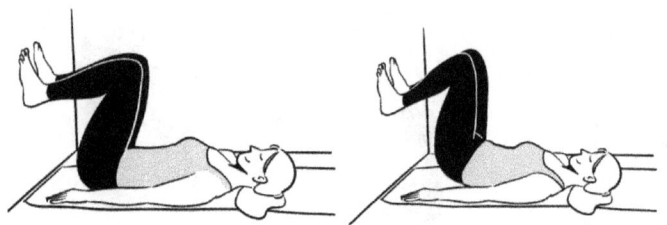

Wall Shoulder Bridge
Works: Core, Lower Body
Benefits: Strength, Balance, Mobility

Lie on your back with your knees bent, feet flat on the floor and hip-width apart. The the tips of your toes should be touching the wall. Flex your glutes and curl your hips under to lift them into the air. Hold for ten seconds and return to the floor. Depending on your strength level, repeat five to 10 times.

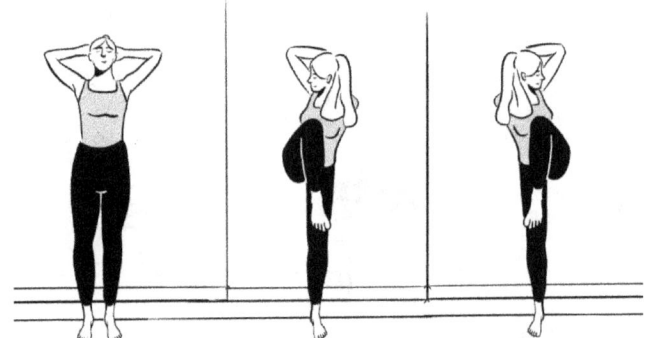

Standing Bike/Crunch
Works: Core, Abs, Spine
Benefits: Cardio, Strength, Balance

Stand with your back to the wall and your feet about six inches away. Bend your elbows and lock your fingers behind your head. Bend your left elbow down towards your right knee while simultaneously bending your right knee up towards your left elbow. Quickly switch sides by next bending your RIGHT elbow down towards your LEFT knee while lifting the knee towards your right elbow. That's one rep. Repeat quickly for 5-10 repetitions. Rest for three breaths then repeat for 5-10 more repetitions. Relax.

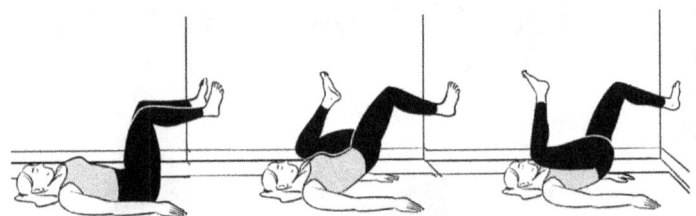

Lifted Knee Tucks
Works: Core, Glutes, Hamstrings
Benefits: Balance, Coordination, Strength & Mobility

Lay on your back with your buttocks about three feet from the wall, your arms at your side, palms on the floor. Bend your knees and place your feet flat on the wall. Use your arms and left foot to elevate your buttocks off the floor while bringing you right knee towards your head. Hold briefly and repeat. Do this ten times and repeat on the opposite side. You can also alternate legs between repetitions.

This marks the end of the exercises for day 18. See you tomorrow.

Day 19. Today we'll focus on balance and stability.

Multi-Stretch

Works: Spine, Hip Flexors, Hamstrings, Glutes, Obliques
Benefits: Flexibility, Mobility, Core

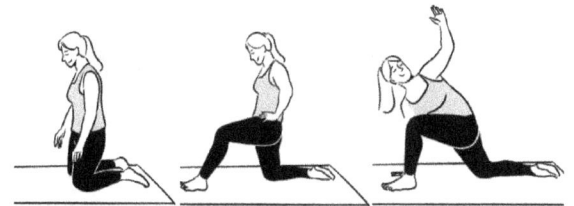

Start on your knees parallel to the wall. Stretch your left leg out in front of you with your leg bent and the foot flat on the floor; basically, you are kneeling on one knee. Lean forward with your torso to add a stretch to the hip flexor. Place one hand on the floor opposite to the front foot. Finally, reach your left arm up and rotate towards the ceiling leading with your upper back and shoulders. Hold for three seconds then repeat on the opposite side.

Hip Flexor Stretch with Chair

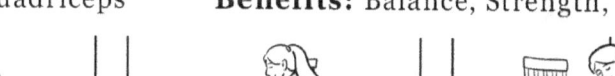

Works: Hip Flexor, Back, Quadriceps   **Benefits:** Balance, Strength, Mobility

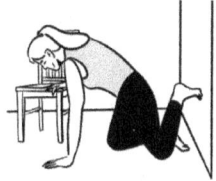 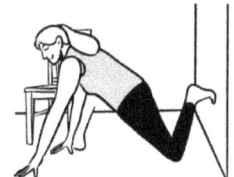 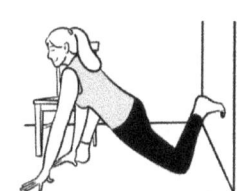 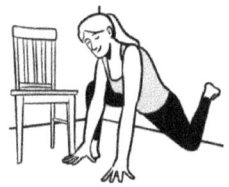

With a chair sideways in front of you, kneel down with your back to and your feet touching the wall. Lean forward so your right hand is on the chair seat for support and your left hand is on the floor. Place your left foot on the wall so that the toes are curled under with the ball of your foot touching. While supporting yourself with the chair, bring your right foot forward and bend your knee so that the foot is flat on the floor. Next, put your right hand on the floor and push your pelvis forward and away from the wall to feel the stretch. Hold for 3-5 seconds and then slightly twist your hips and pelvis to the right as you lift your head. Hold until you feel the muscles loosen (about 10 seconds). Unwind and repeat with the opposite leg on the wall.

The Frog

Works: Knees, Hips, Quads, Groin
Benefits: Strength & Balance

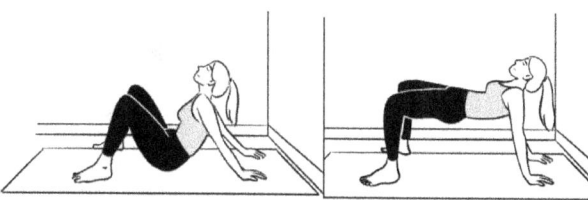

Start in a tabletop or "crab walk" position: Your head, stomach and pelvis pointed towards the ceiling with your feet flat on the floor, knees bent and your hands behind you with your palms on the floor. Keep your arms fully extended and not bent. From here, push your buttocks up to straighten your back and stretch your spine as much as possible. Do these three to five times.

Day 19

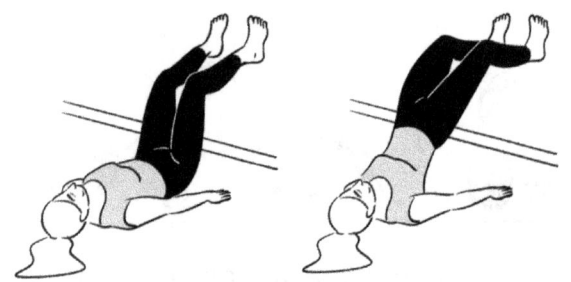

Elevated Glute Bridge
Works: Glutes, Abs, Hamstrings, Hip Flexors
Benefits: Balance, Coordination, Strength, Mobility

Lie faceup and place your feet flat on the wall about hip-width apart with your knees and hips bent at 90-degree angles and your arms along your sides. Lift your hips until your body makes a straight line from your knees to your shoulders. Squeeze your glutes, hold, then lower back to the floor. Repeat 10 times total.

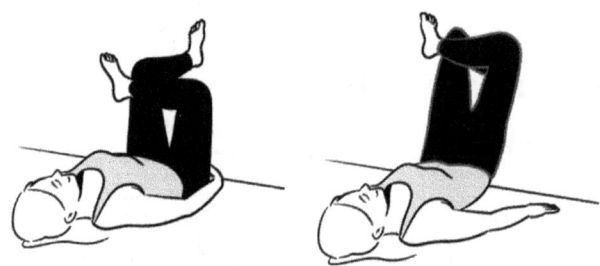

Glute Bridge Cross
Works: Glutes, Abs, Hamstrings, Hip Flexors
Benefits: Balance, Coordination, Strength, Mobility

Lie on your back with your buttocks about a foot from the wall, your feet flat on the wall with your lower legs straight, your knees bent at a 90-degree angle, and your back flat on the mat. Cross your right leg over your left, with your right ankle on your left knee. Raise your buttocks about two feet and hold briefly before lowering back to the mat. Repeat five times for each side.

Marching Glute Bridge

Works: Glutes, Abs, Hamstrings, Hip Flexors   **Benefits:** Balance, Coordination, Strength, Mobility

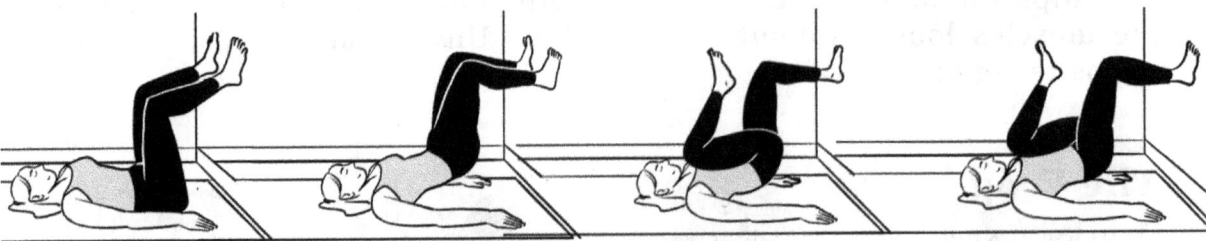

Lie on your back with your buttocks about a foot or so from the wall, your feet flat on the wall so that your lower legs are straight and your knees are bent at a 90-degree angle. Make sure your back is flat against the mat and your arms are along your sides. Lift your hips off the floor and bend your right knee towards your head while keeping your left foot on the wall. Put your right foot back on the wall and bend your left knee, lifting your left foot towards your head. That's one. Repeat 5-10 times.

Day 19

The Hundred
Works: Cardio, Core, Abs
Benefits: Strength, Balance, Cardio

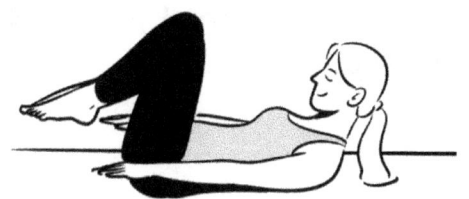

(Intermediate Level) Lie on your back with your knees bent and pointed slightly toward your head and the bottom of your feet parallel to floor. Elevate your arms to a 45-degree angle, in line with your thighs. Then, lift your neck and shoulders off the mat, squeezing your upper abs. Pump your arms as you inhale and exhale slowly. Aim for a total of 100 pumps.

This marks the end of "Day 19" exercises.

Day 20: Alternate Exercises & Rest

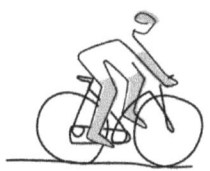 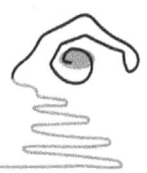 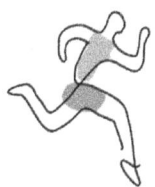 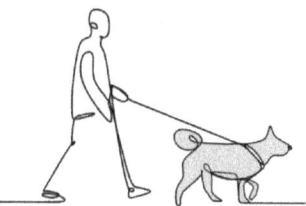

Today, take a break from Wall Pilates and enjoy an alternate exercise on your own such as brisk walking, swimming, or biking. You can also do some of the simple stretching and breathing exercises from earlier chapters in the book. We've included instructions for two basic breathing exercises below.

Belly Breathing
Benefits: Breath Control, Concentration

To start, sit comfortably with your back straight. Place one hand on your chest and the other on your belly. Breathe in deeply through the nose, allowing your belly to expand while keeping your chest still. Hold momentarily and then exhale slowly through your mouth. Continue for about two minutes.

Box Breathing
Benefits: Stress Relief & Discipline

Inhale through the nose slowly while counting to four in your head. Hold that breath for a count of four. Exhale through the mouth for a count of four. Hold that breath out for another count of four. Complete 5-10 cycles.

Day 21. As we move into our third week, if you find any routine too difficult, feel free to modify it, substitute a different exercise, or repeat the previous day's routine until you feel comfortable moving forward. Now, let's get started.

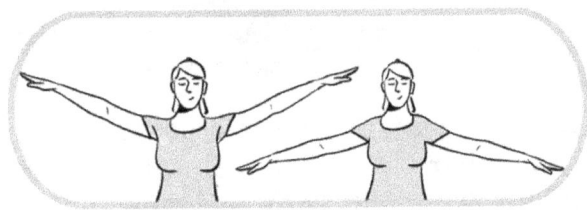

Arm Rolls
Works: Upper Back, Shoulders
Benefits: Warm-Up, Stretch, Cardio

Stand about three feet from the wall, legs about shoulder length apart and your arms out like an airplane. Keeping your elbows locked, make large, forward circles with your hands at medium speed. Do this five times then switch directions for five more repetitions. Repeat in each direction five times.

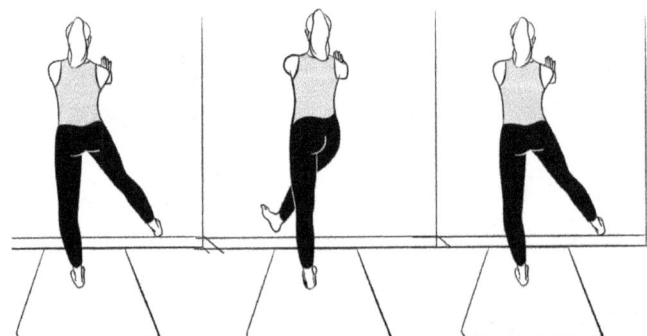

Lateral Leg Swings
Works: Hips, Glutes, Legs
Benefits: Strength, Balance

Lean in from a bit more than an arm's length away and place your palms on the wall. Inhale then exhale as you swing your right leg laterally in front of your left leg towards your left side. Inhale as you return. Keep your legs and knees straight, and avoid twisting your hips. Do this ten times then repeat with the left leg.

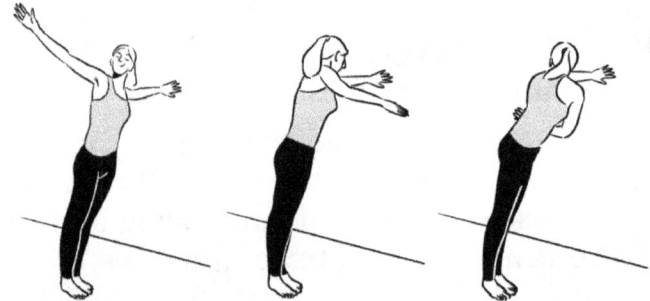

Reach-Twist-Wrap
Works: Chest, Arms, Spine
Benefits: Strength, Fitness

Stand an arm's length away from wall, facing parallel to it. Bend your left arm, lean your body and place your forearm against the wall while keeping your side straight. Reach your right arm out to your side and slightly up and hold briefly as you inhale. Exhale and twist your body to the left while bringing your right arm down and under the left arm while keeping it extended and away from you to "wrap" your body. Repeat 3-5 times on each side.

Day 21

Wall Hands
Works: Back, Chest, Shoulders
Benefits: Flexibility, Warm-Up

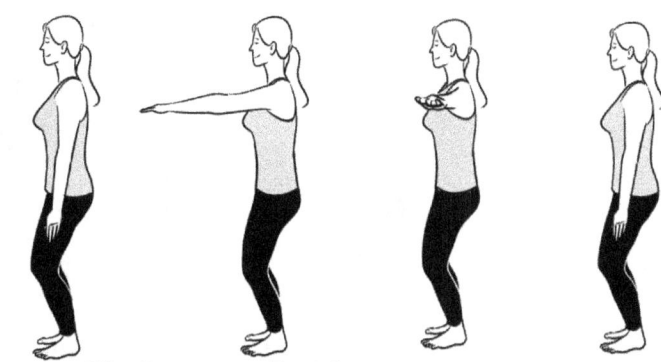

Start with your back against the wall. In one fluid motion, inhale as you raise your arms straight out in front of you with your elbows locked, exhale then up over your head, out to your sides like an airplane and then down. That's one circle. Do five slow "circles" in each direction.

Cactus Arms
Works: Back, Chest, Shoulders
Benefits: Flexibility, Warm-Up

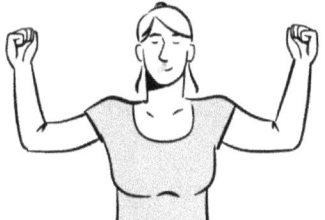 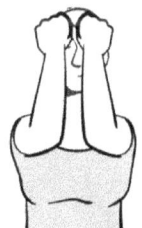

Start with your back and body against the wall. Extend your arms straight out from your sides and bend up at the elbow at a 90-degree angle like a cactus. The back of your hands and forearms should be touching the wall. With arms still bent, move them forward so that your palms and forearms come together in front of you. Hold for three seconds. With elbows still bent, move your arms back so your forearms and outer hands tap the wall. Hold for three seconds. Repeat 15-20 times.

Ankle Circles
Works: Ankles, Calves
Benefits: Flexibility, Warm-Up

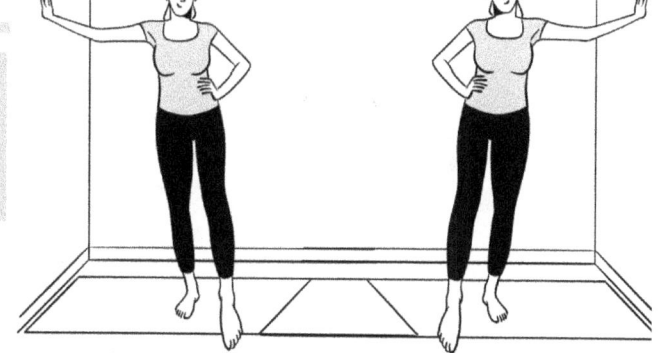

With one hand on the wall for support, lift one foot at at time and make circles with your feet while keeping your leg straight. First in a clockwise direction and then in a counterclockwise direction. Repeat ten times in each direction and two times with each foot.

Day 21

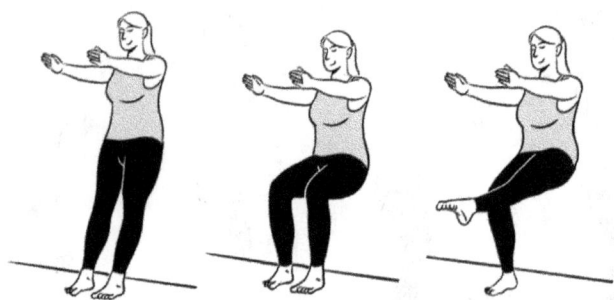

Wall Sit/Leg Out
Works: Quads, Hamstrings, Glutes
Benefits: Balance, Strength, Fitness

Stand with your back on the wall and your feet shoulder-width apart. Hold your hands out in front of you for balance. Bend your knees, lowering your hips deeply so your thighs are parallel with the floor, keeping weight back in your heels. Slowly raise your right leg out so that it is straight with your toes pointed. Hold for 30 seconds. Rise back up and repeat the motion, this time raising the right leg. Relax.

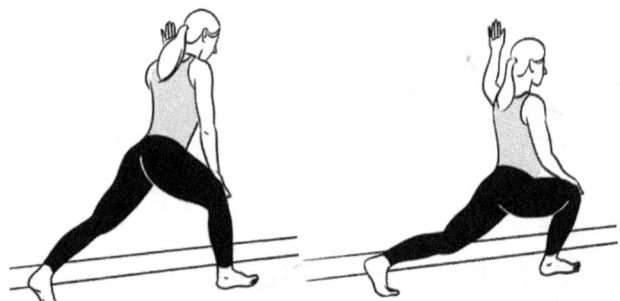

Wall-Supported Lunge
Works: Quads, Hamstrings, Glutes
Benefits: Cardio, Strength, Balance

Stand next to the wall an arm's length away looking down the wall. Place your left hand on the wall and your right hand on your hips knee, or side. Keeping your hips square, bend your right knee as you slide your left leg back behind you into a lunge position, bringing the knee down close to the floor. Hold momentarily, then press the left foot to pull you back to your original position. Repeat five times on each side.

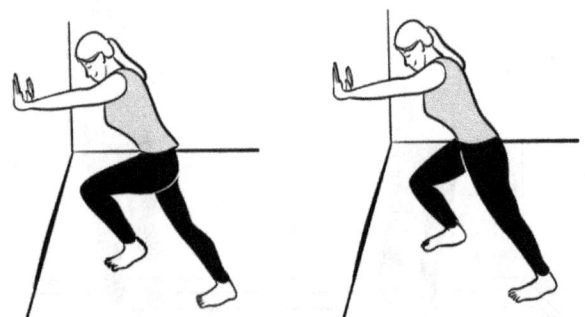

Standing Wall March
Works: Hips, Quads, Glutes
Benefits: Flexibility, Mobility, Balance, Strength

This exercise should mimic a sprint. To start, face the wall about one and a half arm's lengths away. Bend your right leg and lift your knee up quickly and bring back down as you switch to the opposite leg and do the same motion. The faster you switch, the more "cardio" the exercise is. One "set" is 10-15 back-and-forth "march" motions between legs. Do two or three sets, resting for 10 seconds between each.

Day 21

Bear Sequence

Works: Arms, Shoulders, Hips, Calves, Core   **Benefits:** Balance, Strength, Coordination

These five moves should flow one to the other and all begin with the same starting position: like a bear on all fours with your back straight. This is the "basic position". Go through the entire sequence, pausing between each exercise if necessary.

Balance Bear: From the basic position, lift your right hand and your left foot off the floor an inch or two, then replace. Repeat with other side: lift your left hand and your right foot off the floor an inch or two then replace. That's one repetition. Do a total of five to ten repetitions, or "reps", before moving on.

Bear Sequence

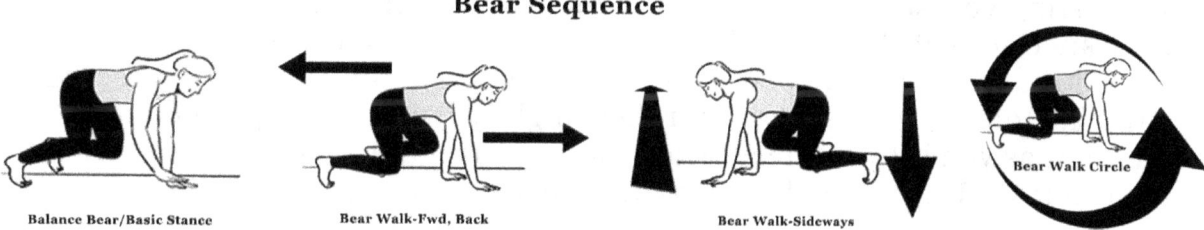

Balance Bear/Basic Stance   Bear Walk-Fwd, Back   Bear Walk-Sideways   Bear Walk Circle

Bear Walk/Forward & Backwards: From the basic position, slowly walk across the floor in the balance bear stance then walk backwards back to your starting position. Repeat once.

Bear Walk/Sideways: From the basic position, walk sideways across the floor in the balance bear stance then sideways back to your starting position. Repeat once.

Bear Walk/Circle: From the basic position, turn around in a circle, first clockwise then counter-clockwise. Repeat once.

Half Windmill Sit

Works: Back, Arms, Shoulders, Waist, Spine
Benefits: Warm-Up, Strength

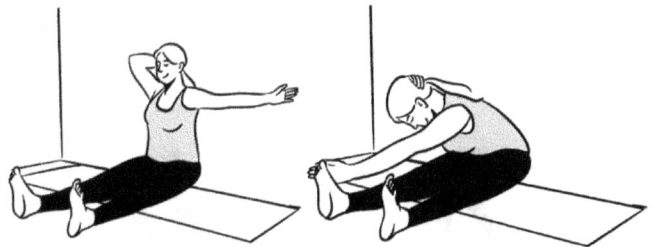

Sit on the floor with your back to the wall and your arms straight out like an airplane with your palms facing out. Bend your elbow to place your right hand on the back of your head. Swing your left arm around to the outside of your RIGHT knee and keeping your back straight, bend to put the back of your left hand on the outside of your right foot. Hold for five seconds then back to the neutral position. Repeat on the opposite side and five times total.

This marks the end of the exercises for day 21.

Day 22. Let's start today with a chair for a prop.

Hip Flexor Stretch

Works: Hips, Back, Quads, Core   **Benefits:** Balance, Mobility, Flexibility

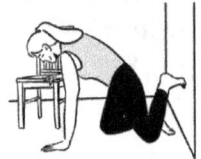 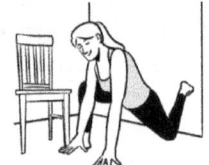 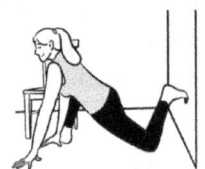 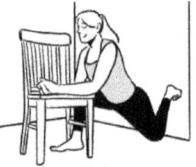

With a chair sideways in front of you, kneel down with your back to and your feet touching the wall. Lean forward so your right hand is on the chair seat for support and your left hand is on the floor. Place your left foot on the wall so that the toes are curled under with the ball of your foot touching. While supporting yourself with the chair, bring your right foot forward and bend your knee so that the foot is flat on the floor. Next, put your right hand on the floor and push your pelvis forward and away from the wall to feel the stretch. Hold for 3-5 seconds and then slightly twist your hips and pelvis to the right as you lift your head. Hold until you feel the muscles loosen (about 10 seconds). Unwind and repeat with the opposite leg on the wall.

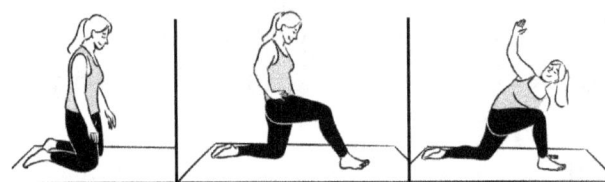

Multi-Stretch
Works: Spine, Hip Flexors, Glutes, Hamstrings, Obliques
Benefits: Flexibility, Mobility

Start on your knees parallel to the wall. Stretch your left leg out in front of you with your leg bent and the foot flat on the floor. Lean forward with your torso to add a stretch to the planted knee's hip flexor. Place one hand on the floor opposite to the front foot. Finally, reach your left arm up and rotate towards the ceiling leading with your upper back and shoulders. Hold for 3 seconds then repeat on the opposite side.

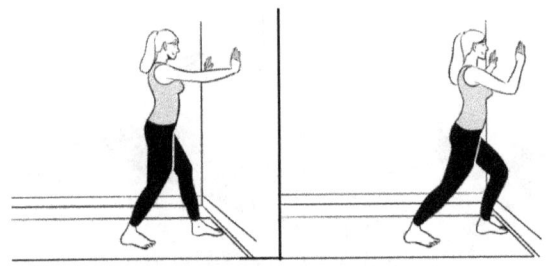

Wall-Facing Lunge
Works: Quads, Hamstring, Glutes
Benefits: Balance, Mobility, Cardio

Put your palms on the wall in front of you. Step your left foot forward until your toes nearly touch the wall and move your right foot backwards. Inhale and bend both knees as you bring the left knee close to the wall and your forearms near the wall. The movement should be slow and fluid. Hold for five seconds and repeat with the opposite leg and side. That's one repetition. Do 10 reps.

Day 22

Lunge-Twist

Works: Legs, Hips, Back, Spine
Benefits: Cardio, Strength, Mobility

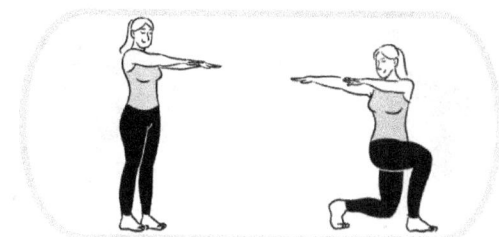

Stand three feet from the wall facing away with your arms extended in front. Bend your left leg backward so that your foot touches the wall. Then, lunge and squat forward with your right leg while twisting your torso to the right. Hold briefly and return to a standing position. Repeat five times then change to the left side. Bend your right leg backward so that your foot touches the wall while bending your left leg out as you lunge forward and twist your torso to the left. Hold briefly and return to a standing position.

Hip Slides

Works: Core, Lower Body
Benefits: Cardio, Strength, Balance

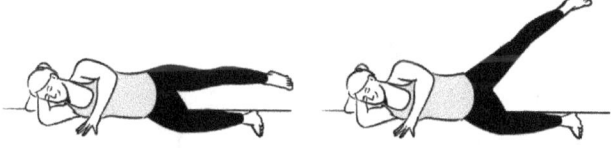

Lie on your side parallel to and facing away from the wall. Both knees should be straight and your top heel on the wall. Raise your top leg along the wall as high as you can, keeping your heel pressed against the wall. Hold briefly then lower. Do this five times then repeat for the opposite side and leg.

The Hundred

Works: Core, Abs, Back, Shoulders
Benefits: Energy, Strength, Balance

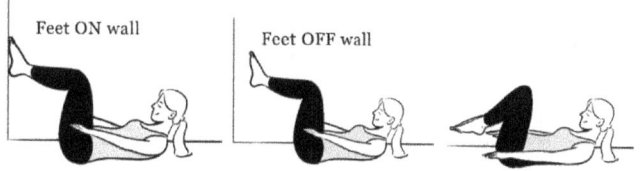

(Beginner) Lie on your back with your knees bent and your feet flat on the wall. Your shins should be parallel to the floor and your thighs should be perpendicular to it. Elevate your arms to a 45-degree angle, in line with your thighs. Then lift your neck and shoulders off the mat, contracting your upper abdominals. Pump your arms as you inhale and exhale slowly. Aim for a total of 100 pumps.
(Intermediate) Same action, but start with your knees bent so your shins are parallel with the floor and your thighs perpendicular to it. Your feet should be in the air parallel to, but not touching the wall. Aim for a total of 100 pumps.
(Advanced) Same action, but start with your feet off the wall, your knees bent and pointed slightly toward your head and the bottom of your feet parallel to floor. Aim for a total of 100 pumps.

Day 22

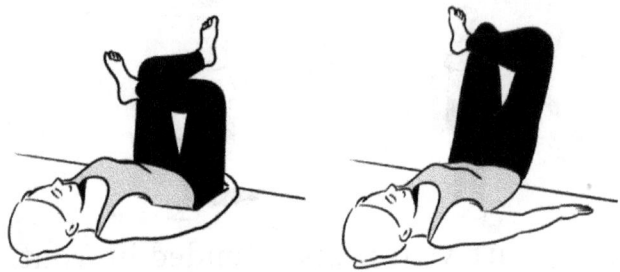

Glute Bridge Cross
Works: Core, Glutes, Hamstrings, Abs, Hips
Benefits: Balance, Strength. Mobility

Lie on your back with your buttocks about a foot or so from the wall, your feet flat on the wall so that your lower legs are straight and your knees are bent at a 90-degree angle. Make sure your back is flat against the mat. Cross your right leg over your left, putting your right ankle on your left knee. Raise buttocks in a glute bridge position and hold for two seconds, then lower to mat. Repeat five times for each side.

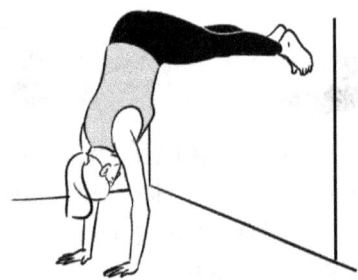

Wall Pike
Works: Arms, Chest, Back, Core
Benefits: Strength, Balance, Mobility

Kneel with your back to the wall and your hands on the floor shoulder width apart. Put your feet on the wall behind you about 3 feet high. Keeping your feet on the wall, lower your upper body to the floor slowly and hold briefly. Push back up to starting position. Repeat 10 times.

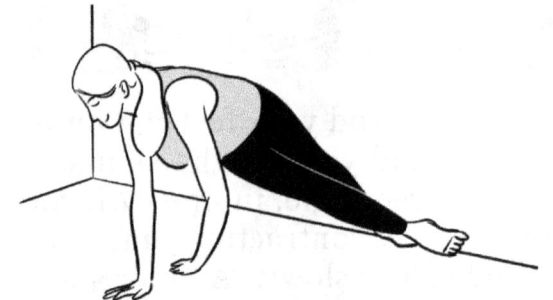

Thread the Needle
Works Chest, Shoulders, Triceps, Core
Benefits: Strength, Circulation, Fitness

Start on your belly in the push-up position. Place your feet in the crevice between the wall and floor with your left toes touching your right heel. Lift your left arm to the ceiling and then rotate your torso to bring your left arm slowly back down between your chest and the floor. Repeat five times then switch sides. Place your right foot behind your left with your toes touching your left heel. Lift your right arm to the ceiling and then rotate your torso to bring your arm slowly back down between your chest and the floor. Repeat five times.

Day 22

Cat-Cow
Works: Spine, Shoulders, Back
Benefits: Mobility, Flexibility

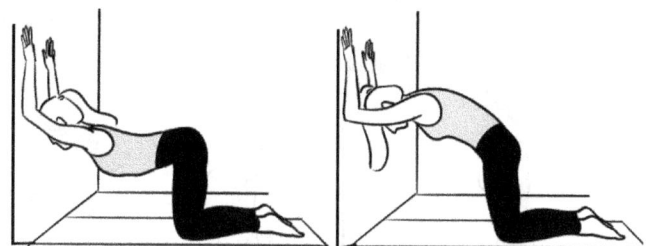

Start on your hands and knees facing the wall about an arm's length away. Lean into the wall and put your elbows, forearms and palms on the wall while arching your back. Hold for three seconds while inhaling and exhaling, then roll your back down while sticking your buttocks out. your back should now be in a simi "U" shape. Hold for five seconds while you inhale and exhale then return to start. Repeat five to ten times focusing on your breathing and form.

Butterfly
Works: Hamstricngs, Quads, Groin
Benefits: Flexibility, Mobility, Warm-Up

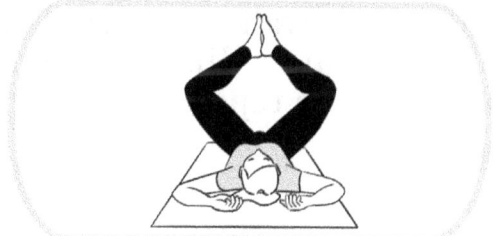

Lie on your back with your feet and hips against the wall. Bend your elbows and let your arms rest above your head on the mat. Keeping your feet on the wall, bend your knees in toward your chest while lowering your heels as low as you can and putting the soles of your feet together. Stay in this position for two to three minutes.

The Scoop
Works: Shoulders, Chest, Spine, Core
Benefits: Posture, Flexibility, Breathing

This is a great starting or finishing exercise and stretch, or for morning wake-ups to start your day. I also like to use one or two reps of this exercise between others in my routine to get the oxygen flowing.With your arms straight down interlock your fingers with your palms facing up. Inhale deeply as you bring your interlocked palms towards your chin. Turn your interlocked palms outward and exhale slowly as you straighten your elbows until your arms are fully extended in front of you. Keep the motion going as you raise your interlocked hands above your head with your palms towards the ceiling. Hold momentarily, and then release your hands and bring them slowly to your sides. Repeat five times.

This marks the end of the exercises for day 22.

Day 23: Starting with Warm-Ups.

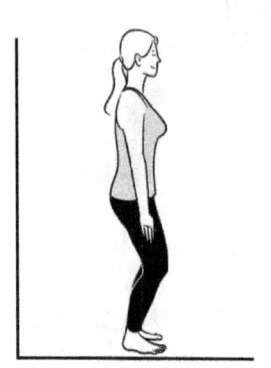 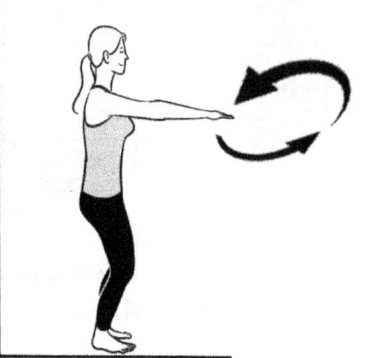

Arm Circles in Front
Works: Shoulders, Upper Back
Benefits: Flexibility, Balance, Cardio

Stand about three feet from the wall, legs about shoulder length apart and knees bent slightly. Extend your arms out in front of you like you're sleepwalking. Keeping your elbows locked, make circles with your arms at medium speed. Do this five times then switch directions for five more repetitions. Repeat in each direction three times.

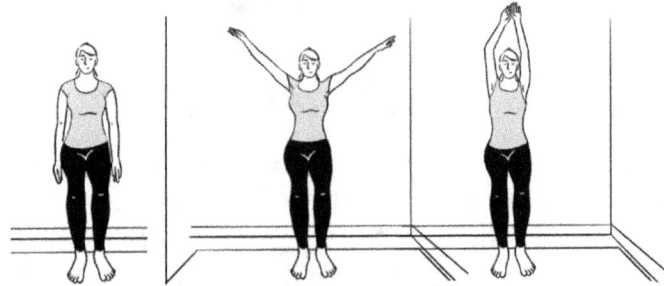

Arm Slides
Works: Shoulders, upper Back
Benefits: Flexibility, Strength

Standing with your back to the wall, bend your knees as you walk your feet out about an arm's length out in front of you while keeping your back and buttocks on the wall into a partial wall sit position. Keeping your elbows locked, slide your arms straight up above your head until your hands meet. Hold momentarily and then bring them back down. That's one. Repeat for ten total repetitions.

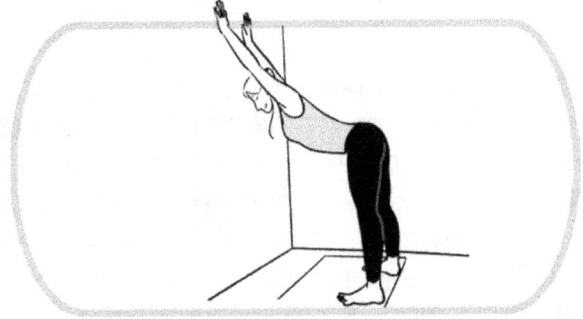

Arms Overhead
Works: Chest, Shulders, Upper Back
Benefits: Flexibility & Strength

Stand facing the wall, an arm's length away. Raise your arms over your head and place your palms flat against the wall. Keeping your arms straight, lean forward and press your chest towards the wall until you feel a stretch in your upper chest. Hold the stretch for 20-30 seconds, then relax and repeat.

Day 23 Main Exercises

Lateral Raises

Works: Deltoids, Upper Back
Benefits: Cardio, Strength

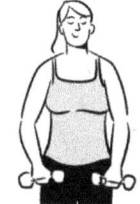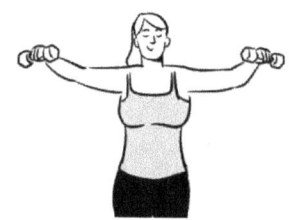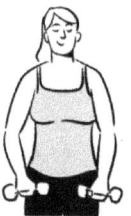

Start with empty hands and add weights as it gets easier. You can use anything you have around the house to start: Canned goods are great for beginners. Just make sure you have the same weight in each hand. To Start, stand upright with your arms bent at the elbows. Bring both elbows straight up to shoulder level as if pouring water out of a pitcher. Bring back to start and repeat. Do this 6-10 times. Increase weight as you get stronger.

Reach-Twist-Wrap

Works: Legs, Shoulders, Core
Benefits: Balance, Coordination, Stability, Strength, Mobility

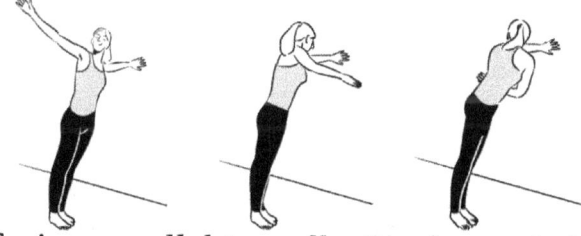

Start an arm's length away from wall, facing parallel to wall. Bend your left arm and place forearm against wall keeping your side straight. Extend your right arm out and slightly up and hold briefly. Twist your body to the left while bringing right arm down and under the left arm while keeping it extended and away from the body to "wrap" your body. Inhale as you reach and exhale as you wrap. Repeat 3-5 times and then switch sides.

Kneeling Archer

Works: Thoracic spine, Rhomboids, Trapezius   **Benefits:** Stability, Flexibility, Strength

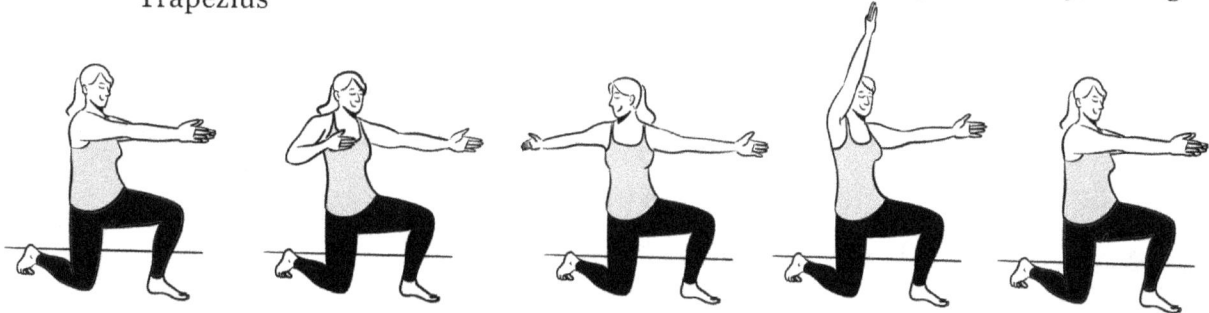

Start by kneeling down on your right knee and your right leg bent so your foot is flat on the floor. Extend your arms in front of you with your palms together. Keep your left arm still as you pull your right arm straight back and rotate your torso while extending your right arm behind you and, in a circular motion, raise your right arm over your head and down in front of you to join the other palm. Repeat three times before switching sides.

Day 23

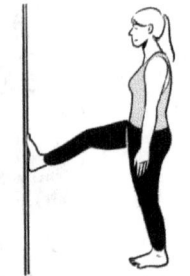
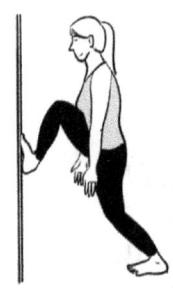

Press Lunge
Works: Hips, Quads, Ankles
Benefits: Balance, Stability, Strength, Fitness

Stand one leg-length away from the wall and place your right foot on the wall at hip-height, leaving your left leg straight. Bend your right knee and lunge forward until your knee is pointed up, keeping your upper body upright. Pause briefly, then press through your foot to return to your starting position. Repeat ten times then switch sides.

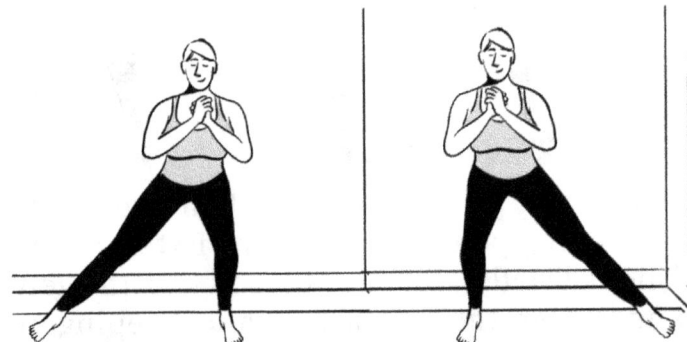

Standing Side Lunge
Works: Quads, Glutes, Hamstrings, Adductors & Abductors
Benefits: Balance, Stability, Strength

With your back to wall clasp your hands in front of you and bend your elbows. Slide your left foot to the left and bend your left knee while keeping your right leg straight and in place on the floor. Hold momentarily and return to center. Repeat on the opposite side by bending and sliding your righ foot while keeping your left foot in place. That's one repetition. Do five to ten repetitions.

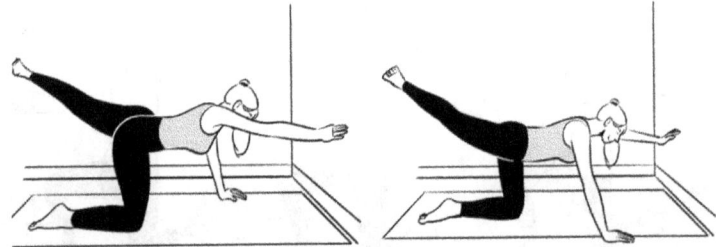

Tabletop Reach
Works: Shoulders, Hips, Glutes, Core
Benefits: Flexibility & Strength

Start on your hands and knees facing the wall about an arm's length away. Extend your left leg straight back with toes pointed straight as you simultaneously reach out to the wall with your right hand. Return to neutral position and then extend your right leg out as you touch the wall with your left hand. Do this in rapid, but smooth succession five to ten times, alternating sides each time.

Day 23

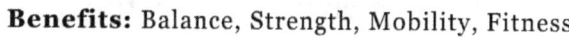
Glue Bridge with Leg Raise

Works: Core, Glutes, Hamstrings, Abs, Upper Back

Benefits: Balance, Strength, Mobility, Fitness

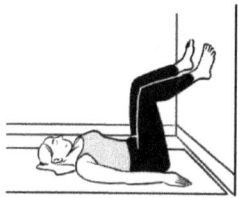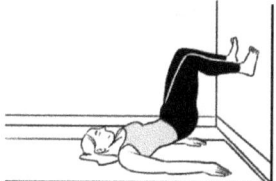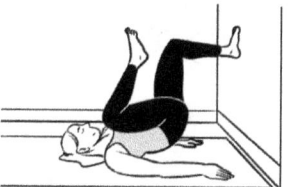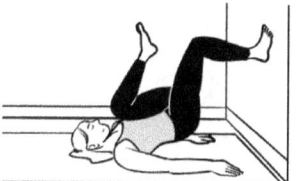

Lie on your back with your feet against the wall. Bend your knees to 90 degrees and extend your arms along your sides. Lift your glutes off the floor and keep them there. Inhale as you raise your left leg up straight in the air and towards your head. Return leg to wall and repeat with the right leg. When raised, your legs should be fully extended, and as close to your head as possible. Keep your head and shoulders on the mat. Repeat the back-and-forth between legs for five to ten repetitions.

Split Stance Deadlift

Works: Glutes, Hamstring, Quads, Core
Benefits: Strength, Balance, Coordination

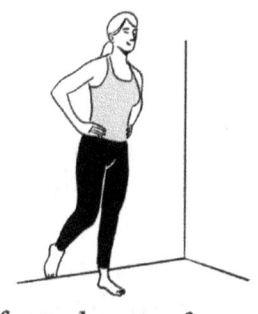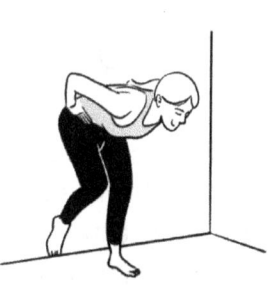

Stand with your back to the wall, both feet about a foot away. Place your right heel behind you on the wall with toes on the floor. With both knees slightly bent, bend at your hips keeping your back flat. Keep your front knee over your front ankle and tighten your core. Once your upper body is about parallel to floor, use your right foot to stand up, extending your hips. Do 8-10 repetitions then switch sides.

Squat with Calf Raise

Works: Calves, Quads, Glutes, Hamstrings
Benefits: Strength, Balance, Coordination

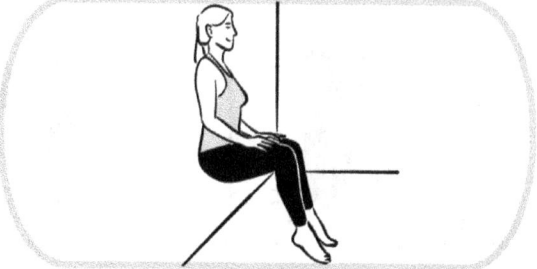

Start with your back against the wall and your feet shoulder-length apart. Squat down until your upper legs are parallel with the floor and hold. Lift your heels off the ground. Hold briefly then return your heel to the floor, and push up out of the squat. Repeat 5-10 times.

This marks the end of our exercises for day 23.

Day 24: Alternate exercises and rest.

Today you can take a rest from Wall Pilates and enjoy an alternate exercise on your own such as brisk walking, swimming, or biking. You can also do some of the simple stretching and breathing exercises from earlier chapters in the book.

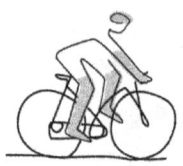 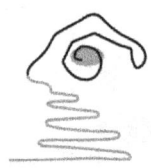 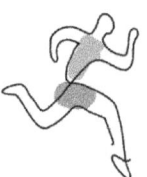 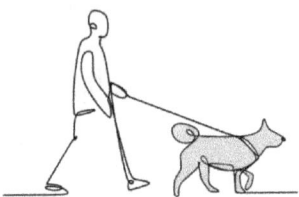

Day 25

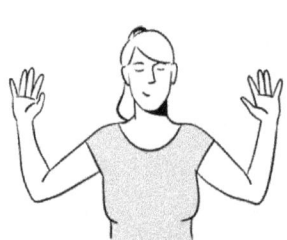

Wall Angels
Works: Back, Neck, Shoulders
Benefits: Flexibility, Mobility, Strength

Stand with your back to the wall and feet about six inches away. Bend your arms 90 degrees while keeping them as flat against the wall as possible. Keep your back and arms on the wall as you slowly raise your arms up oer your head. Use your abs to press your back against the wall. Hold momentarily at the top and bring back down to the starting position. Repeat five to ten times.

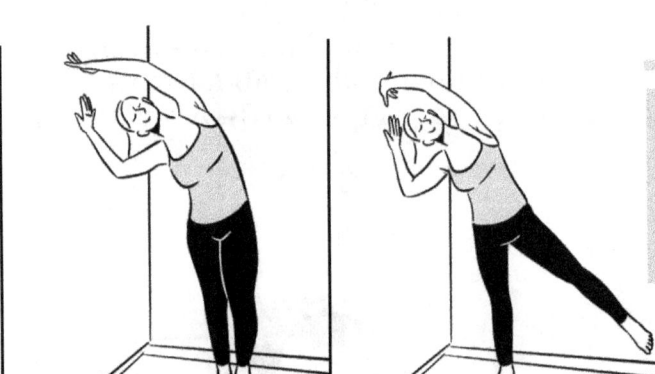

Side Bend with Leg Lift
Works: Obliques, Inner Thigh, Glutes, Hips, Groin
Benefits: Mobility, Flexibility

Begin by standing sideways and an arm's length from the wall, with your right side closest to the wall and feet hip-width apart. Put your right palm on the wall, extend your left arm overhead, and slide your right hand down the wall as you bend your torso to the right attempting to touch the wall. Hold this position and lift your left leg up and out sideways for ten repetitions. Return to neutral then switch sides and repeat.

Day 25

Single Leg Circles

Works: Quads, Hamstrings, Groin
Benefits: Cardio, Strength, Balance

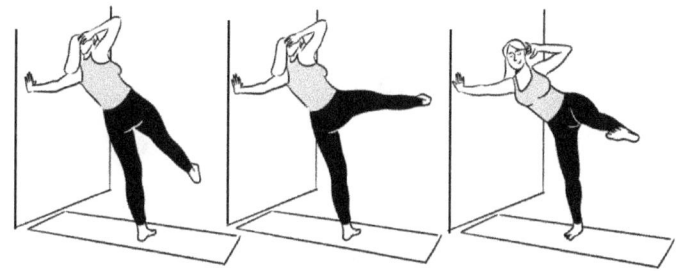

Standing next to the wall, bend slightly towards it at the hips and place your left hand on the wall. Bend your right elbow and put your right hand on the back of your head. Keeping your left leg and back straight, make a wide sweeping circle that goes in front, beside and behind you as much as possible. Do five circles in each direction then switch legs.

Bear Squat

Works: Legs, Shoulders, Core
Benefits: Balance, Coordination, Stability, Strength, Mobility

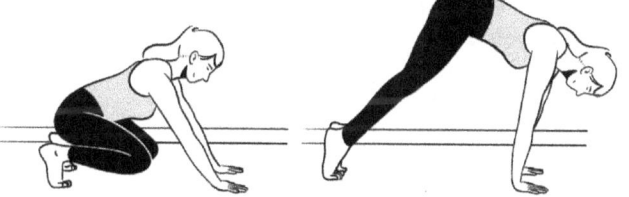

Start on all fours (hands and feet) with your shins parallel with the floor. Bend your knees and lower your buttocks to touch your heels. Then quickly explode up and forward, straightening your legs and lifting your hips toward the sky as you shift your weight over your hands. At this point, your body should be an inverted "V" with your toes and palms touching the floor. Hold momentarily and repeat the action from the start. Do 5-10 repetitions.

Kneeling Archer

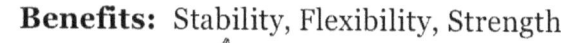

Works: Thoracic spine, Rhomboids, Trapezius   **Benefits:** Stability, Flexibility, Strength

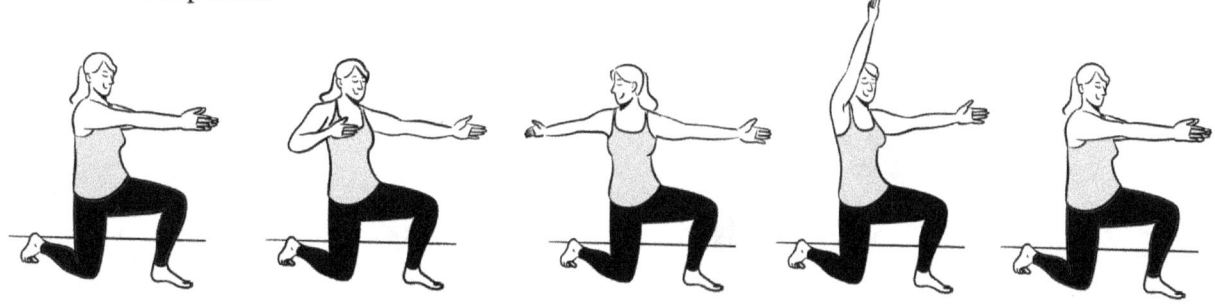

Start by kneeling down on your right knee and your right leg bent so your foot is flat on the floor. Extend your arms in front of you with your palms together. Keep your left arm still as you pull your right arm straight back and rotate your torso while extending your right arm behind you and, in a circular motion, raise your right arm over your head and down in front of you to join the other palm. Repeat three times before switching sides.

Day 25

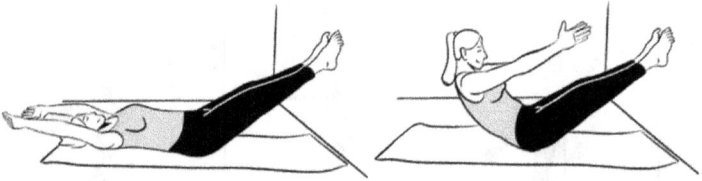

Wall Teaser
Works: Abs, Back, Shoulders
Benefits: Strength, Control

This one is more difficult than it looks! Sit on the floor with your feet on the wall to form a slight "V". Inhale as you slowly roll your body up and move your hands and arms towards your feet until your eyes are level with your toes. Do not bounce and make sure to keep your feet on the wall. Hold for a count of five and then back to the floor. Repeat five times.

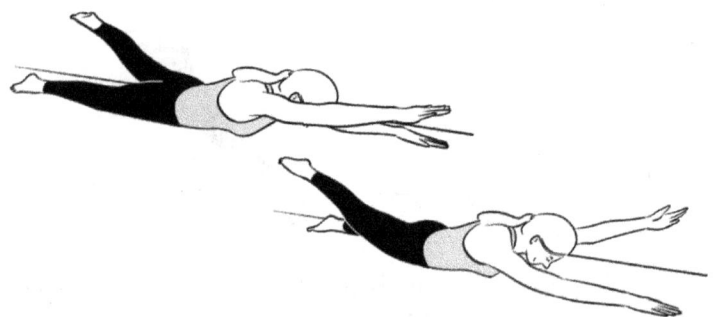

Swimmer Reach
Works: Abs, Shoulders, Hips
Benefits: Strength, Flexibility

Laying face-down on a mat parallel to the wall, stretch your legs behind you and your arms above your head with palms on the mat. Your head can be up or resting on the mat. Breathe in and raise your locked right arm and locked left leg straight up at the same time while keeping them parallel to the floor. Hold momentarily and breathe out as you return them to the mat. Repeat with the left arm and right leg. Breathe in and raise your left arm and right leg straight up at the same time while keeping them parallel to the floor. Lift both up as much as possible and hold before returning to the mat. Repeat five times on each side, alternating sides each time. Try and stretch your legs out and reach your arms as much as possible as you perform the movements.

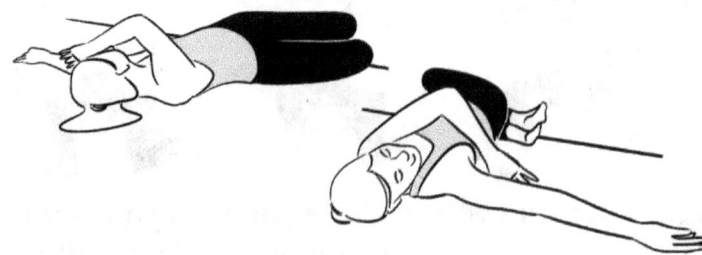

Torso Twist on Mat
Works: Spine, Shoulders, Back
Benefits: Strength, Flexibility

Lie on your back with your feet touching the wall for reference. Bend your legs at the knees slightly and rotate them to the right so your knees touch the mat. At the same time, bend your arms across your body to the left, touching the mat with your hands. Hold for 10 seconds and repeat on the opposite sides.

Day 25

Chest Lift
Works: Back, Spine
Benefits: Balance, Posture, Coordination

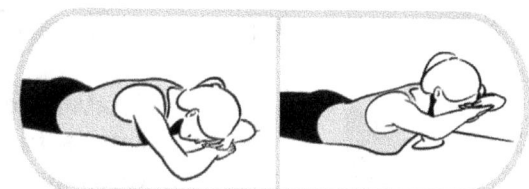

Lay face-down the floor with your elbows bent and your forehead resting on your hands. Breathe in, and as you breathe out, bend at the waist as you lift your arms, head and torso off the mat as far as possible. Hold momentarily and bring back to starting position. Repeat five to ten times.

Child's Pose
Works: Legs, Back, Shoulders
Benefits: Flexibility, Mobility, Strength

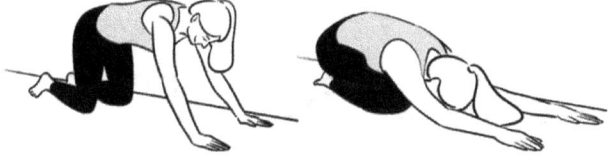

On your hands and knees with your arms out slightly in front of you, fold back, bending your knees and folding your body so that your legs are underneath you. Stretch out your arms with your palms on the floor. Hold 30 seconds then repeat.

The Frog
Works: Knees, Hips, Groin, Glutes
Benefits: Balance, Coordination, Stability

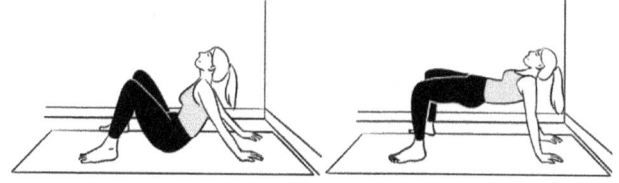

Start in a "crab walk" position: Your head, stomach and pelvis pointed towards the ceiling with your feet flat on the floor, knees bent and your hands behind you with your palms on the floor. Keep your arms fully extended and not bent. From here, push your buttocks up to straighten your back and stretch your spine as much as possible. Do this three to five times.

The Hundred

Works: Thoracic spine, Rhomboids, Trapezius **Benefits:** Stability, Flexibility, Strength

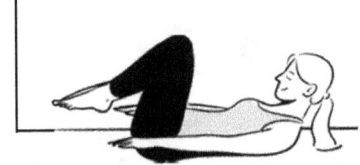

(Advanced Level) Lie on your back with your knees bent and and pointed slightly toward your head and the bottom of your feet parallel to floor. Raise your arms to a 45-degree angle, lift your head and shoulders off the mat, and pump your arms rapidly as you inhale and exhale slowly. Repeat until you reach a total of 100 arm pumps.

Side Step Against Wall

Works: Groin, Adductors, Quads, Glutes **Benefits:** Stability, Mobility, Strength

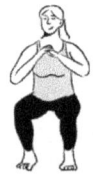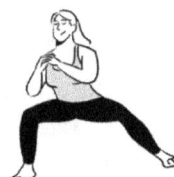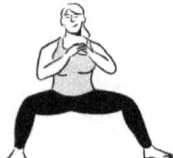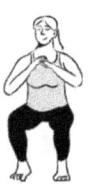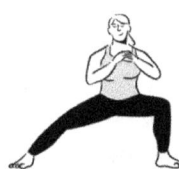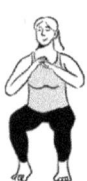

Walking sideways against a wall in a squat position. Start with your back against the wall and your knees bent. Bend your elbows and clasp your hands in front of you. Slde your left foot and leg away from your right foot while keeping your body in the same position. Immediately bring your right foot and the rest of your body to the left back towards the other foot and leg so that you are again in a wall squat-your original position. Do this for five steps to the left and then five steps back to the right. Rest momentarily and then repeat in both directions once more.

Standing Bicycle

Works: Back, Hip Flexors, Abs **Benefits:** Strength, Flexibility, Balance

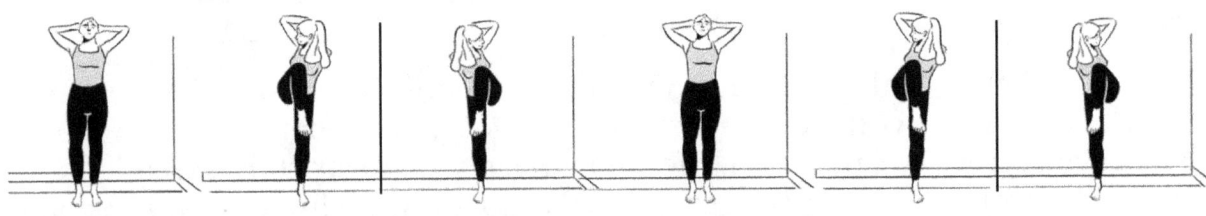

Stand with your back to the wall and your feet about six inches away. With your fingers locked behind your head, bend your torso, head and left elbow down towards your right knee while simultaneously bending your right knee up towards your left elbow. Quickly switch sides by next bending your torso, head and RIGHT elbow down towards your LEFT knee while lifting the knee towards your right elbow. Repeat quickly 10 times. Rest for 30 seconds then repeat for three more sets.

Day 26

Bird Flap
Works: Scapula, Chest, Shoulders
Benefits: Flexibility, Balance, Cardio

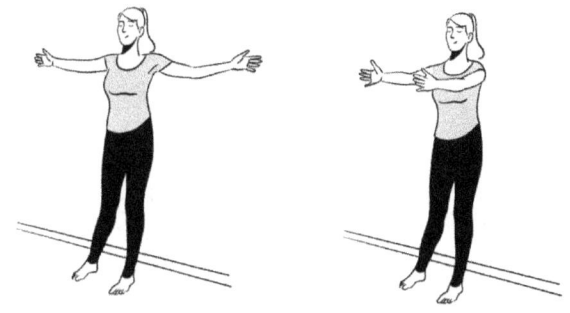

Stand with you back to the wall, glutes and shoulders touching. Your feet should be about two feet away. Spread your arms straight out like an airplane, with the backs of your arms and hands touching the wall and your palms facing out. Keeping your elbows locked, bring your arms straight out in front of you so that your thumbs are up and your palms are facing each other and nearly touching. Hold momentarily and then return your arms to the wall. Repeat at a medium speed 15 times and two sets.

Wall Push-Up
Works: Chest, Shoulders, Upper Back
Benefits: Mobility, Posture, Strength

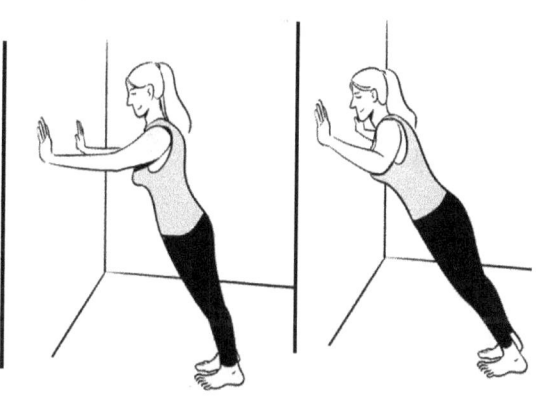

Standing about an arm's length away from the wall, lean in and put your palms flat on the wall, slightly wider than shoulder-width apart, with your arms straight, and your fingers pointing up. Keeping your spine straight, slowly bend your arms until your head touches the wall. Pause. Slowly push yourself away from the wall and back up. That's one. Do this 10-15 times for two sets.

Russian Twist
Works: Hips. Core, Abs, Spine
Benefits: Flexibility, Mobility, Balance, Cardio

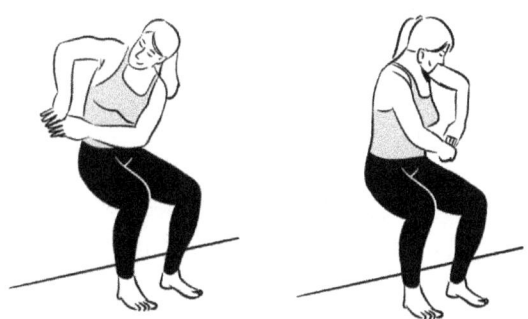

Stand with your knees bent and your back against the wall in as simi-squat position. Quickly twist your torso to the left while reaching your arms across your body to touch the wall on your left with your hands. Twist your torso back to the right, reaching your arms across your body to touch the wall on your right with your hands. Quickly repeat this side-to-side motion for 15 to 20 sets of twists. Repeat once more if desired.

Day 26

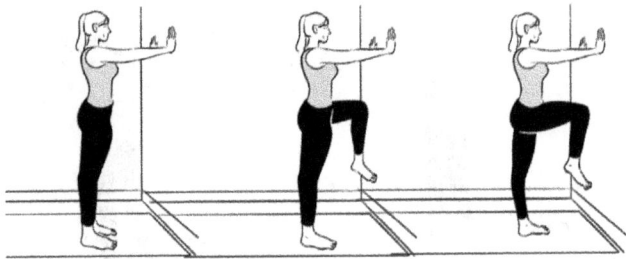

Mountain Climber
Works: Core, Abs, Hips
Benefits: Flexibility, Mobility, Balance

This movement is one that imitates quickly climbing up a steep hill. Stand an arm's length away with your hands on the wall and your arms fully extended but not bent. Bend your leg and lift your right knee towards the wall with your toes and lower leg pointed down. Immediately return to start and repeat with the left leg, while keeping your back straight. The movements should be controlled, but quick. Do two sets of 10-15 repetitions each and rest in between.

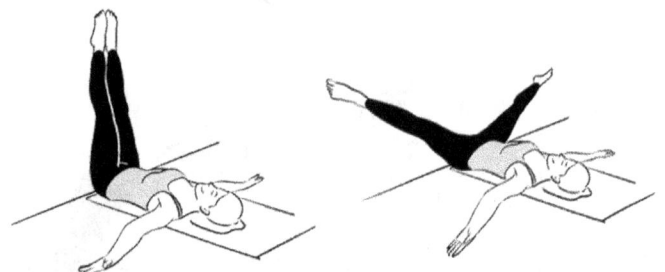

Wall Scissors
Works: Abs, Glutes, Inner Thighs
Benefits: Flexibility, Mobility, Balance, Strength

Lay on your side with your legs bent and against the wall. Roll over onto your back so that your legs and buttocks are up against the wall. Stretch your arms out from your side like an airplane. Open your legs widely to stretch the inner thigh and hold for two seconds. Bring back to neutral. Repeat 10 times.

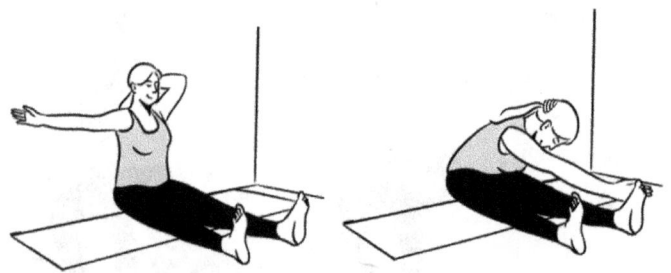

Half Windmill Sit
Works: Back, Waist, Spine
Benefits: Strength, Flexibility

Sit on the floor with your back to the wall and your arms straight out like an airplane with your palms facing out. Bend your elbow to place your right hand on the back of your head. Swing your left arm around to the outside of your RIGHT knee and keeping your back straight, bend to put the back of your left hand on the outside of your right foot. Hold for five seconds then back to the neutral position. Repeat on the opposite side and five times total.

Day 26

Wall Hip Slides
Works: Core, Lower Body
Benefits: Mobility, Cardio, Strength

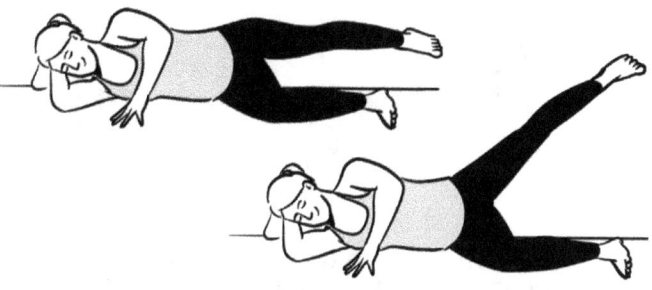

Lie on your side parallel to and facing away from the wall. Both knees should be straight and your top heel should be on the wall. If you want, put a towel between your heel and the wall for smoother movement. Raise your top leg along the wall as high as you can, keeping your heel pressed against the wall. Hold briefly, then lower. Do this five times then switch to the opposite side and leg for a total of two times each side.

Glute Bridge Cross
Works: Abs, Glutes, Hip Flexors
Benefits: Strength, Balance, Mobility

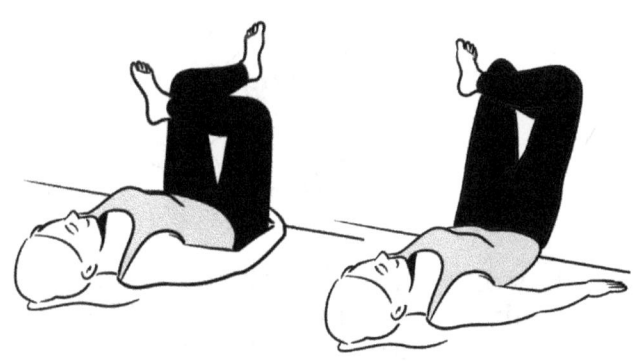

Lie on your back with your buttocks about a foot or so from the wall, your feet flat on the wall so that your lower legs are straight and your knees are bent at a 90-degree angle. Make sure your back is flat against the mat. Cross your right leg over your left, putting your right ankle on your left knee. Raise buttocks in a glute bridge position and hold for two seconds, then lower to mat. Repeat five times for each side.

Marching Glute Bridge

Works: Abs, Glutes, Hamstrings, Hip Flexors **Benefits:** Cardio, Strength, Balance, Mobility

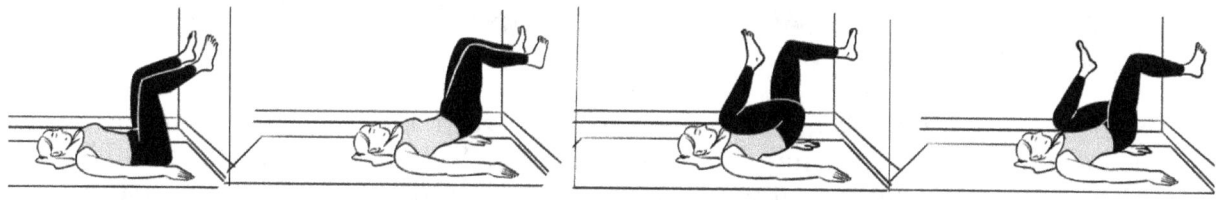

Start where the previous exercise left off: on your back with your buttocks about a foot or so from the wall, your feet flat on the wall so that your lower legs are straight and your knees are bent at a 90-degree angle. Make sure your back is flat against the mat and your arms are along your sides. Lift your hips off the floor and bend your right knee towards your head while keeping your left foot on the wall. Put your right foot back on the wall and bend your left knee, lifting your left foot towards your head. That's one. Repeat 5-10 times.

Day 26

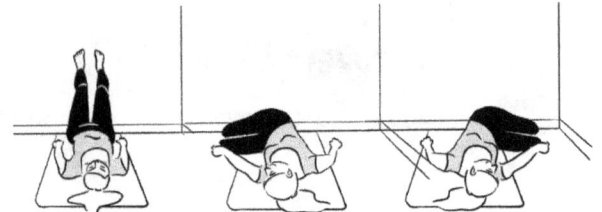

Knee Rolls

Works: Hips, Back, Glutes, Abs
Benefits: Cardio, Strength, Mobility

Start on your back with your arms to your side, knees bent and your feet flat on the wall for spacing. Bring your knees toward your chest slightly and roll your legs to the left until they touch the floor. Hold momentarily and then roll them back to the right until they touch the floor on the right. That's one. Repeat five to ten times. For a more difficult exercise, perform with legs almost straight.

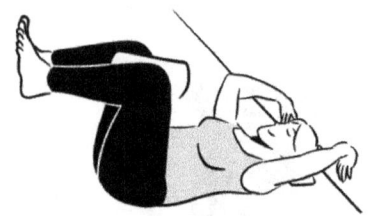

Reverse Crunch

Works: Abs, Glutes, Inner Thighs
Benefits: Flexibility, Mobility, Balance, Strength

Lay on your back with your arms over your head and your palms pressed against the wall. Lift your hips off the ground, bringing your knees toward your chest. Lower your legs back down without touching the floor. Complete three sets of 15 reps.

Side Step Against the Wall

Works: Quads, Glutes, Hamstrings, Adductors, Abductors

Benefits: Cardio, Balance, Mobility

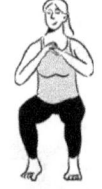 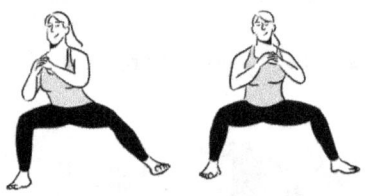 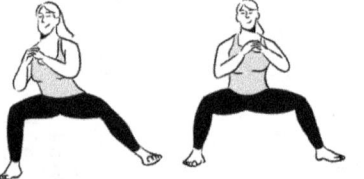

Start with your back against the wall and your knees bent. Bend your elbows and clasp your hands in front of you. Slide your left foot and leg away from your right foot while keeping your body in the same position. Immediately bring your right foot and the rest of your body to the left back towards the other foot and leg so that you are again in a wall squat-your original position. Do this quickly for five steps to the left and then five steps back to the right. Rest momentarily and then repeat in both directions once more.

This marks the end of the exercises for day 26.

Day 27. Find your favorite spot and let's go!

Lateral Leg Swings

Works: Hips, Glutes, Lower Body
Benefits: Flexibility, Mobility, Independence, Strength

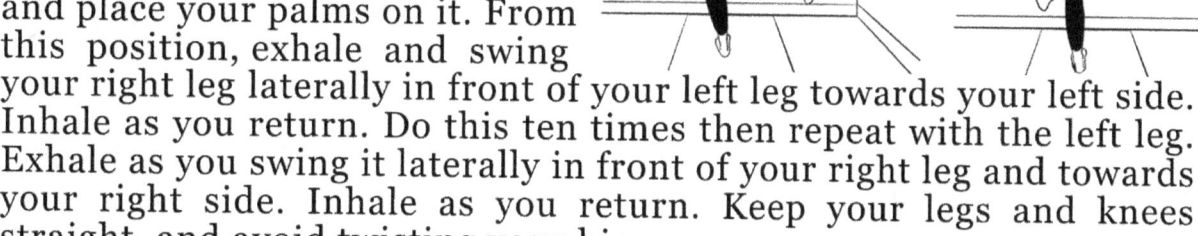

Stand straight in front of the wall and place your palms on it. From this position, exhale and swing your right leg laterally in front of your left leg towards your left side. Inhale as you return. Do this ten times then repeat with the left leg. Exhale as you swing it laterally in front of your right leg and towards your right side. Inhale as you return. Keep your legs and knees straight, and avoid twisting your hips.

Side Leg Lift

Works: Glutes, Hips, Groin
Benefits: Balance, Flexibility, Mobility

Stand sideways, an arm's length from the wall, with your right side closest to the wall and your feet hip-width apart. Put your right forearm on the wall, extend your left arm overhead, and slide your right hand down the wall as you bend your torso to the right. Hold this position while lifting your left leg up and out sideways for ten repetitions. Switch sides and repeat. Do two sets on each side.

Standing Bicycle

Works: Back, Hip Flexors, Abs
Benefits: Strength, Flexibility, Balance

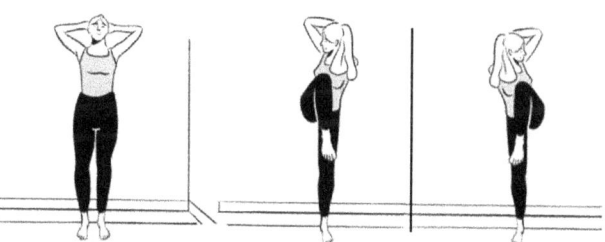

Stand with your back to the wall and your feet about six inches away. Bend your elbows and put your hands behind your head and lock your fingers. Bend your torso, head and left elbow down towards your right knee while simultaneously bending your right knee up towards your left elbow. Quickly switch sides by next bending your torso, head and RIGHT elbow down towards your LEFT knee while lifting the knee towards your right elbow. Repeat quickly 10 times. Rest for 30 seconds then repeat for three more sets.

Day 27

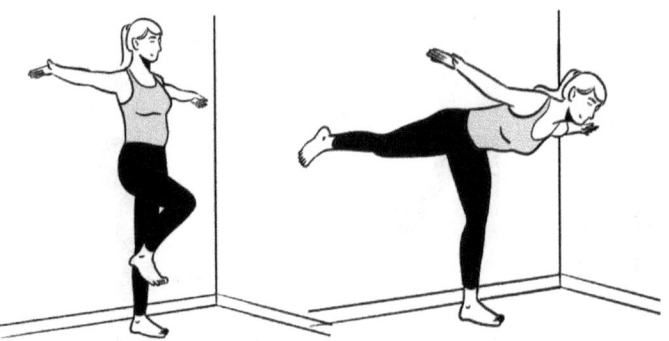

Flying Flamingo
Works: Hips, Glutes, Core, Abs
Benefits: Flexibility, Mobility, Balance, Strength

Stand on your left leg with right knee bent and your right foot next to your left knee. Place your Place your hands on your hips and find your balance. Extend your arms out like an airplane as you pretend that your bent right leg and hips are fused. Hinge forward, moving your right leg rearward and upward. Return to the start. Do five reps on the right side, then switch to having the left foot up while standing on your right leg.

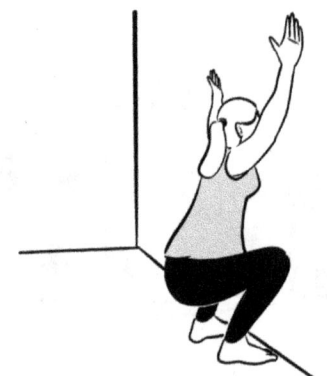

Forward Squat
Works: Ankles, Hipss, Thighs
Benefits: Balance, Mobility, Control

Start facing the wall with your feet shoulder length apart and your toes about a foot from the wall. Keeping your head up, lift your arms above your head and squat down until your thighs are parallel with the floor. Hold for a second, push back up. Repeat 8-10 times. As you get more comfortable, put your feet closer to the wall, but make sure to keep your back straight and your head up.

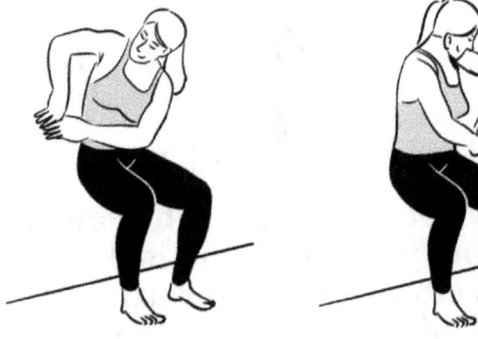

Russian Twist
Works: Hips. Core, Abs, Spine
Benefits: Flexibility, Mobility, Balance, Cardio

Stand with your knees bent and your back against the wall in as simi-squat position. Quickly twist your torso to the left while reaching your arms across your body to touch the wall on your left with your hands. Twist your torso back to the right, reaching your arms across your body to touch the wall on your right with your hands. Quickly repeat this side-to-side motion for 15 to 20 sets of twists. Repeat once more if desired.

Day 27

Cat-Cow

Works: Thoracic spine, Shoulders, Back
Benefits: Flexibility, Mobility Independence, Strength

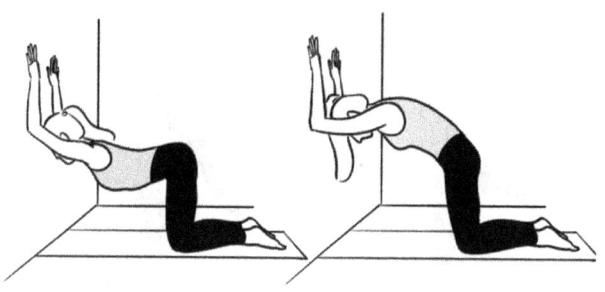

Get on your hands and knees facing the wall about an arm's length away. Lean into the wall and put your elbows forearms, and palms on the wall while arching your back. Hold for a count of five while inhaling and exhaling. Next, roll your back down while sticking your buttocks out. Your back should now be in a simi "U" shape. Hold for five seconds while you inhale and exhale.

Kneeling Archer

Works: Thoracic spine, Rhomboids, Trapezius
Benefits: Stability, Flexibility, Strength

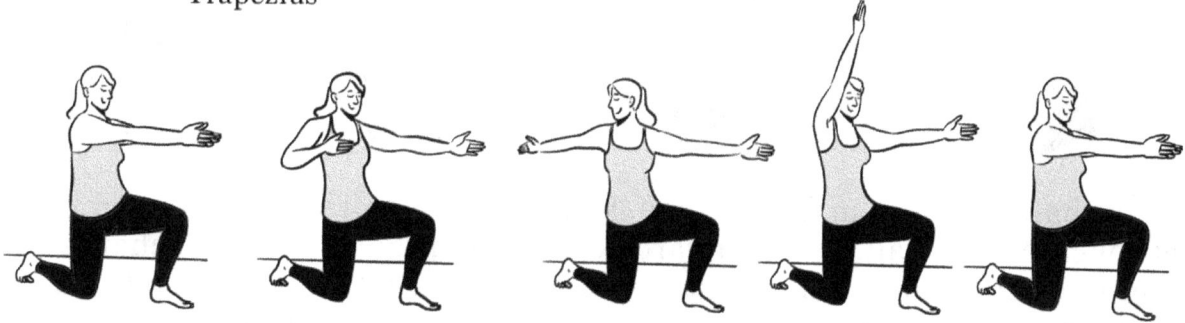

Start by kneeling down on your right knee and your right leg bent so your foot is flat on the floor. Extend your arms in front of you with your palms together. Keep your left arm still as you pull your right arm straight back and rotate your torso while extending your right arm behind you and, in a circular motion, raise your right arm over your head and down in front of you to join the other palm. Repeat three times before switching sides.

Standing Knee Extension

Works: Upper Lats, Abd, Quads
Benefits: Strength, Flexibility, Balance

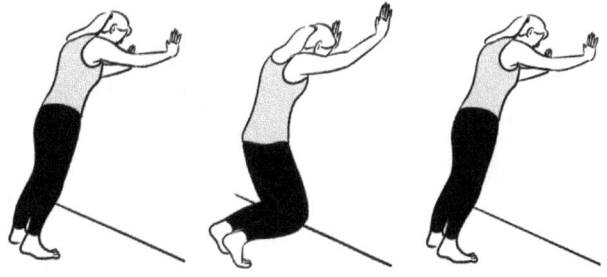

Start by facing the wall about one and a half arm lengths away. Lean over and put your hands on the wall without bending your knees. Keeping your feet in place, slowly bend your knees, hold momentarily, then return to your starting position. Repeat 10 times for two sets with 45 seconds rest in between each.

Day 27

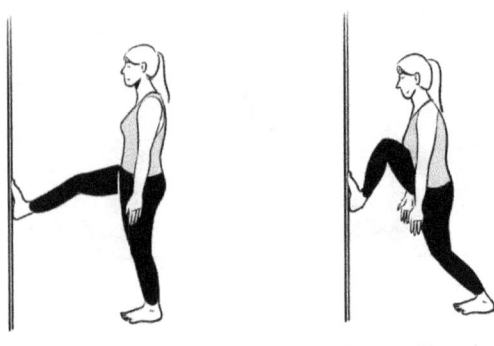

Press Lunge

Works: Knees, Hips, Quads, Glutes
Benefits: Flexibility, Mobility, Balance,

Stand one leg-length away from the wall. Balance yourself, then place your right foot on the wall at hip-height, leaving your left leg straight. Bend your right knee and lunge forward until your knee is pointed up, keeping your upper body neutral and upright. Pause for one second, then press forcefully through the ball of your foot to return to your starting position. Repeat 10 times then switch sides. For a more difficult workout, alternate legs between repetitions.

Hip Flexor Stretch

Works: Hips, Back, Quads, Core   **Benefits:** Balance, Mobility, Flexibility

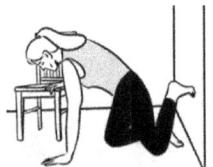 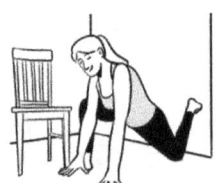 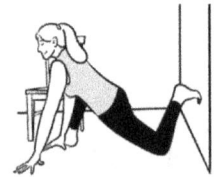 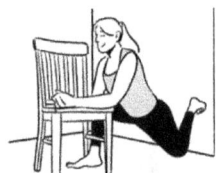

With a chair sideways in front of you, kneel down with your back to and your feet touching the wall. Lean forward so your right hand is on the chair seat for support and your left hand is on the floor. Place your left foot on the wall so that the toes are curled under with the ball of your foot touching. While supporting yourself with the chair, bring your right foot forward and bend your knee so that the foot is flat on the floor. Next, put your right hand on the floor and push your pelvis forward and away from the wall to feel the stretch. Hold for 3-5 seconds and then slightly twist your hips and pelvis to the right as you lift your head. Hold until you feel the muscles loosen (about 10 seconds). Unwind and repeat with the opposite leg on the wall.

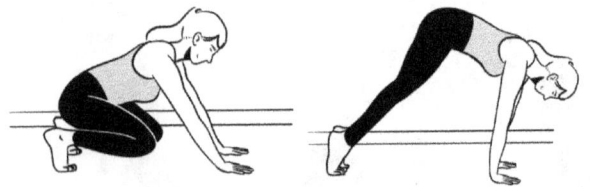

Bear Squat

Works: Hips, Shoulders, Calves, Core
Benefits: Balance, Coordination, Cardio

Start bent over on your hands and toes, then bend your knees and lower your buttocks to touch your heels. Quickly launch yourself up and forward, straightening your legs and lifting your hips up as you shift your weight over your hands. At this point, your body should be an inverted "V" with your toes and palms touching the floor. Hold momentarily then return to start. Do 5-10 repetitions and two sets with 30-45 seconds rest in between each set.

Day 28: The final day of your 28-Day Success Plan! Let's start with some warm-ups.

The Scoop

Works: Shoulders, Chest, Spine, Upper Back
Benefits: Posture, Flexibility, Breathing

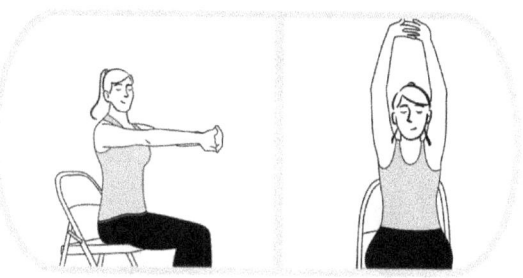

Interlock your fingers and inhale as you bring them towards your chin. Exhale slowly as you straighten your elbows and turn your interlocked palms outward until your arms are fully extended. Keep the motion going as you raise your hands above your head with your palms towards the ceiling. Release your hands, turn your palms out, and bring them slowly to your sides. Repeat five times. Also good for adding between other exercises for extra energy.

Wall Angels

Works: Back, Neck, Shoulders
Benefits: Flexibility, Mobility, Strength

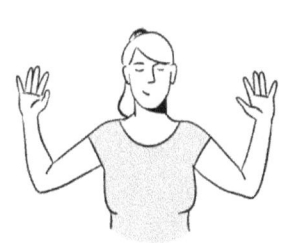 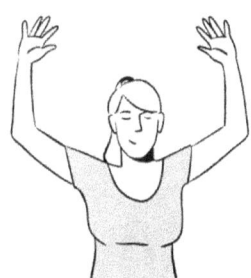

Stand with your back to the wall and feet about six inches away. Bend your arms 90 degrees while keeping them as flat against the wall as possible and slowly raise them arms up as far as possible. Use your abs to press your back against the wall. Hold for three seconds at the top then bring back down. Repeat five times.

Single Arm Pec Stretch

Works: Back, Chest, Shoulders
Benefits: Flexibility, Warm-Up

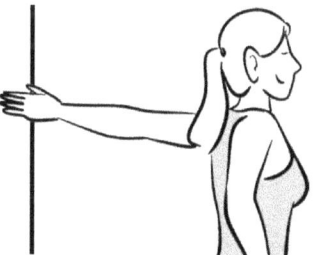 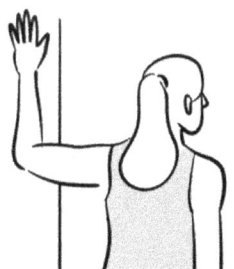

This exercise can be done with your arm extended or bent at the elbow. For arm extended, stand facing the wall an arm's length away. Lift your left arm to shoulder height, place your palm on the wall and twist your body gently to the right. Hold for ten seconds. Focus on feeling a stretch in the chest and shoulders. Repeat the stretch on the opposite side. For bent arm, bend your arm at the elbow, place your forearm and palm against the wall and rotate your body away from the wall.

Day 28

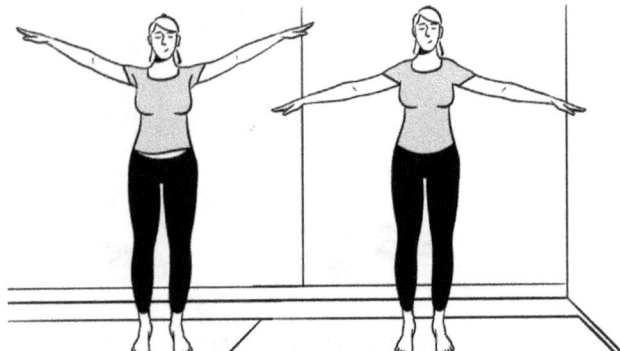

Arm Rolls
Works: Shoulders, Upper Back
Benefits: Flexibility, Warm-Up

Stand about three feet from the wall, legs about shoulder length apart and your arms out like an airplane. Keeping your elbows locked, make large, forward circles with your hands at medium speed. Do this five times then switch directions for five more repetitions. Repeat one time for a total of two sets. Rest for 30-45 seconds in between sets.

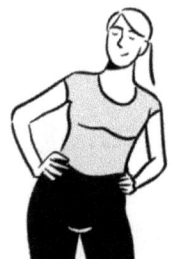 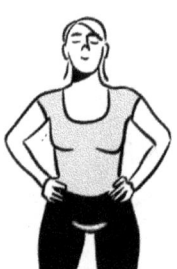 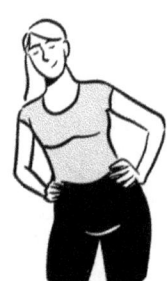

Hip Circles
Works: Hips
Benefits: Flexibility, Mobility

Stand facing the wall, with your feet spread shoulder-width apart and about two feet away from the wall. Put your hands on your hips and pull in your stomach so that you engage your core muscle. Bend to the side slightly as you rotate your hips clockwise 10 times at a medium speed. Repeat in the opposite direction. Gradually increase the size of the circles and the speed of the rotation as you become more flexible and comfortable with the exercise.

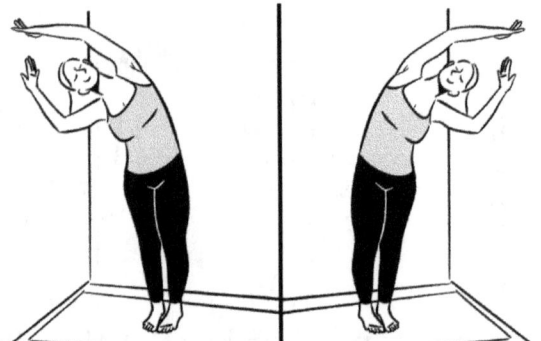

Side Bend/Side Stretch
Works: Hips, Groin, Obliques
Benefits: Mobility, Warm-Up

Begin by standing sideways arm's length from the wall, with your right side closest to the wall and feet hip-width apart. Put your right forearm on the wall, extend your left arm overhead, and slide your right hand down the wall as you bend your torso to the right. Hold this position while lifting your left leg up and out sideways for ten repetitions. Switch sides and repeat.

Day 28

Wall Plank
Works: Triceps, Scapula, Core
Benefits: Strength, Fitness

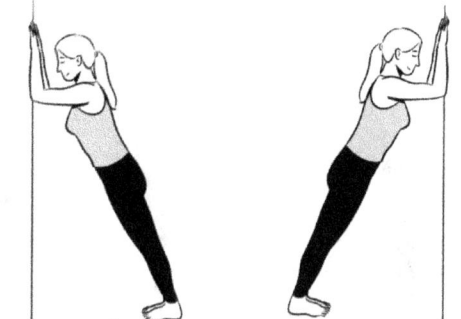

Stand facing the wall about one and a half arm's length away. Lean into the wall, bend your arms and place your forearms and hands on the wall with your palms touching the wall. Hold this position for 30 seconds to two minutes making sure to keep your spine in a straight line. Do not let your hips bend in to the wall!

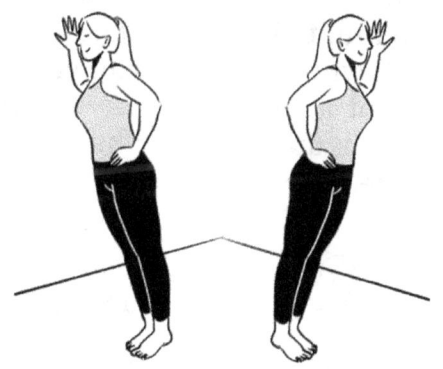

Side Plank
Works: Obliques, Shoulders, Core
Benefits: Warm-Up, Flexibility, Strength

Stand next to the wall and about three feet away. Put your right hand on your right hip and bend your left elbow in a 90-degree angle. Keeping your body straight, lean sideways and place your left forearm on the wall so it's supporting you on the wall. Hold for one minute on each side. Repeat for two sets total.

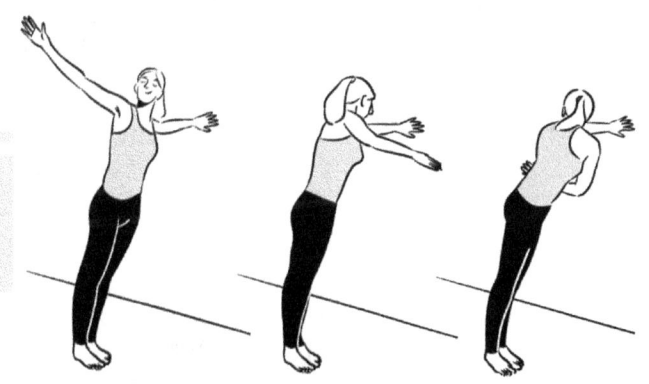

Reach-Twist-Wrap
Works: Legs, Shoulders, Core
Benefits: Balance, Coordination, Stability

Start an arm's length away from wall, facing parallel to wall. Bend left arm and place forearm against wall. The side of your body should be leaning to wall, but straight. Extend your right arm out and slightly up and hold briefly. Twist your body to the left while bringing right arm down and under the left arm while keeping it extended and away from the body to "wrap" your body. Inhale as you reach and exhale as you wrap. Repeat 3-5 times and then switch sides.

Day 28

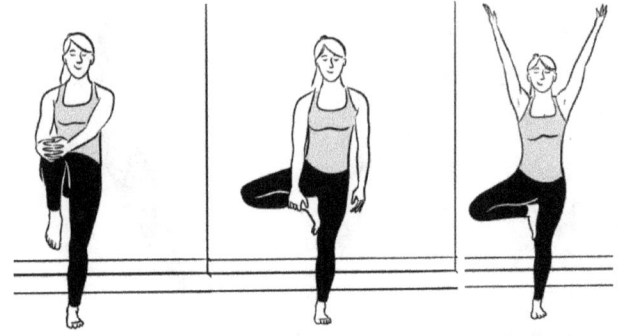

Wall Tree
Works: Legs, Shoulders, Core
Benefits: Balance, Coordination, Flexibility, Pelvic Stability, Core Strength, Upper Body Mobility

For beginners, use the wall for balance. Once you are comfortable with the exercise, do it away from the wall, but close enough for safety. Stand facing away from the wall slightly and bend your right knee, grabbing it with your hands and locking them around it. Pause until you are stable and then grab your right foot with your right hand, twisting it slightly so that the inner thigh is looking upward. Bring it up slowly-as high as you can against your left leg with the bottom of your right foot against the side of your left leg. Lock it in if possible then swing your arms up over your head. Hold for 30-60 seconds, then release. Repeat with the other side.

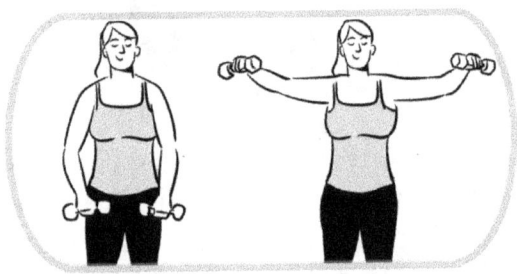

Lateral Raises
Works: Deltoids, Traps, Upper Back
Benefits: Flexibility, Mobility

Weights are optional for beginners. You can use anything you have around the house such as canned goods or hand weights. Just make sure you have the same weight in both hands. Stand upright with your arms bent at the elbows. Bring both elbows straight up to shoulder level as if pouring water out of a pitcher. Bring back to start and repeat. Do this 6-10 times and two sets. Increase weight as you get stronger.

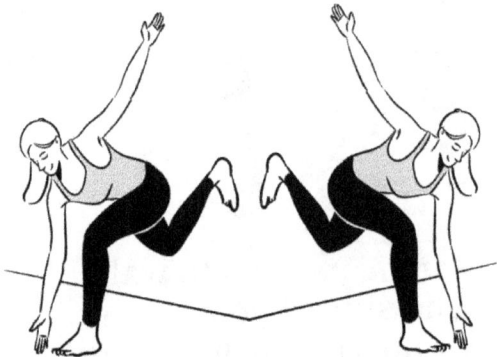

Runner Lunge
Works: Glutes, Quads, Hamstrings
Benefits: Balance, Coordination, Flexibility, Pelvic Stability, Core Strength, Upper Body Mobility

Stand facing away from the wall with back three feet away. Lift your right leg to the wall with toes touching. Bend you left knee deeply and extend your arms like and airplane. Keeping your arms straight, touch your right hand to you the inside of your left foot while twisting your upper body. Hold for three seconds then straighten left leg. Repeat 2-5 times for each side.

Day 28

Reverse Leg Lfts

Works: Hamstring, Spine, Hips
Benefits: Mobility, Balance, Strength

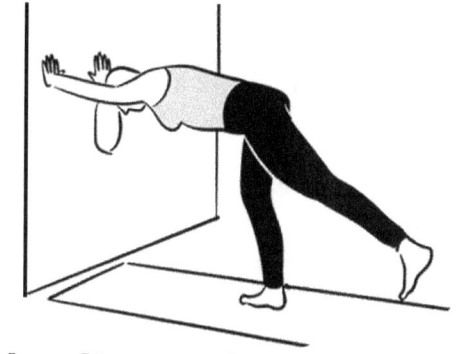

Start by facing the wall a bit more than an arm's length away. Bend at the waist keeping your body straight and put your palms on the wall bending until your body forms an "L". Keeping your hips pointing towards the floor, swing your right leg out behind you and up as far as you comfortably can. Hold for 1 second and bring back to the start position. That's one. Repeat for a total of ten repetitions then switch to the left leg for ten reps.

Cat-Cow

Works: Thoracic spine, Shoulders, Back
Benefits: Stability, Flexibility

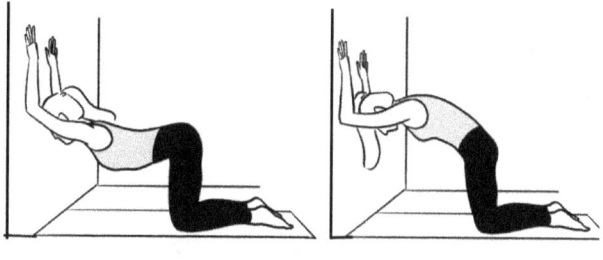

Get on your hands and knees facing the wall about an arm's length away. Lean into the wall and put your elbows, forearms, and palms on the wall while arching your back. Hold for a count of five while inhaling and exhaling. Next, roll your back down while sticking your buttocks out. Your back should now be in a simi "U" shape. Hold for five seconds while you inhale and exhale. Repeat five to seven times.

Half Windmill Sit

Works: Core, Obliques, Hips, Thighs
Benefits: Balance, Coordination, Stability

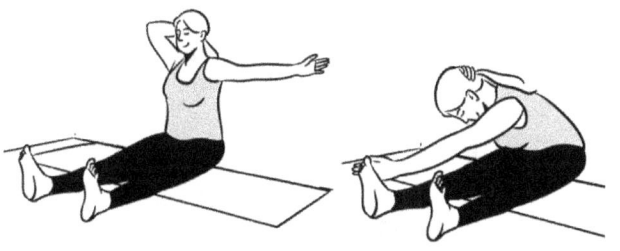

Sit on the floor with your back to the wall and your arms straight out like an airplane. Put your right hand on the back of your head. Keeping your back straight, bend and swing your left arm down to put the back of your left hand on the outside of your right pinky toe. Hold briefly then back to the neutral position. Repeat on the opposite side. That's one rep. Do ten reps each side, rest for 30 seconds then repeat once.

Day 28

The Hundred

Works: Thoracic spine, Rhomboids, Trapezius   **Benefits:** Stability, Flexibility, Strength

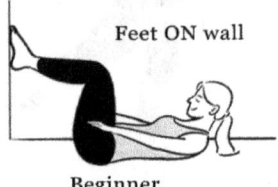
Feet ON wall
Beginner

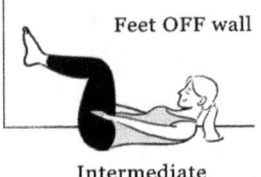
Feet OFF wall
Intermediate

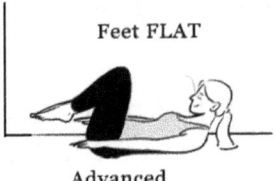
Feet FLAT
Advanced

(Beginner) Lie on your back with your knees bent and your feet flat on the wall. Your shins should be parallel to the floor and your thighs should be perpendicular to it. Elevate your arms to a 45-degree angle, in line with your thighs. Then lift your neck and shoulders off the mat, contracting your upper abdominals. Pump your arms as you inhale and exhale. Aim for 100 pumps.
(Intermediate) Same action, but start with your knees bent so your shins are parallel with the floor and your thighs perpendicular to it. Your feet should be in the air parallel to, but not touching the wall.
(Advanced) Same action, but start with your feet off the wall, your knees bent and pointed slightly toward your head and the bottom of your feet parallel to floor. Aim for a total of 100 pumps.

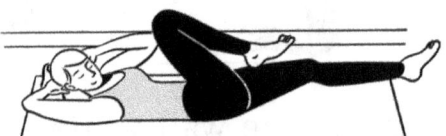

Single Leg Bicycle
Works: Core, Glutes, Hamstrings, Hips
Benefits: Flexibility, Mobility, Balance

Lay on your back with your buttocks about three feet from the wall and your arms at your side, palms on the floor. Bend your knees and place both feet flat on the wall. Use your arms and LEFT foot to elevate your buttocks off the floor while bringing you RIGHT knee towards your head. Hold briefly then repeat with the opposite side. Use your arms and RIGHT foot to elevate your buttocks off the floor while bringing your LEFT knee towards your head. Hold briefly and return. Do this 10 times.

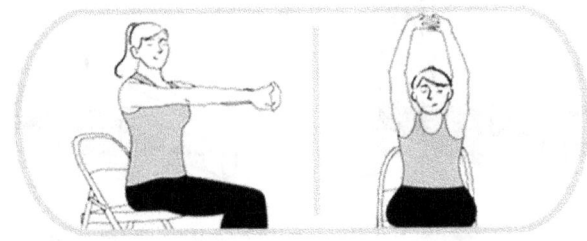

The Scoop
Works: Shoulders, Chest, Spine, Back
Benefits: Posture, Flexibility, Breathing

With your arms straight down interlock your fingers with your palms facing up. Inhale deeply as you bring your interlocked palms towards your chin. Turn your interlocked palms outward and exhale slowly as you straighten your elbows until your arms are fully extended in front of you. Keep the motion going as you raise your interlocked hands above your head with your palms towards the ceiling. Hold momentarily, and then release your hands and bring them slowly to your sides or lap. Do 5 Reps.

Congratulations! You've made it to the end of your 28-Day Success Plan!

The increased energy and sense of vitality you might be feeling are a direct result of your new-found movement. Exercise gets your blood flowing and energizes your body and mind. Keep going by crafting your own routines from upcoming chapters, or go back and run through the plan again, starting with day one. Work your way through the exercises, but change it up by adding repetitions, weights, or resistance bands to make them more challenging. In the next few chapters, we've grouped the exercise routines into chapters by their specific benefits to the body and your fitness goals.

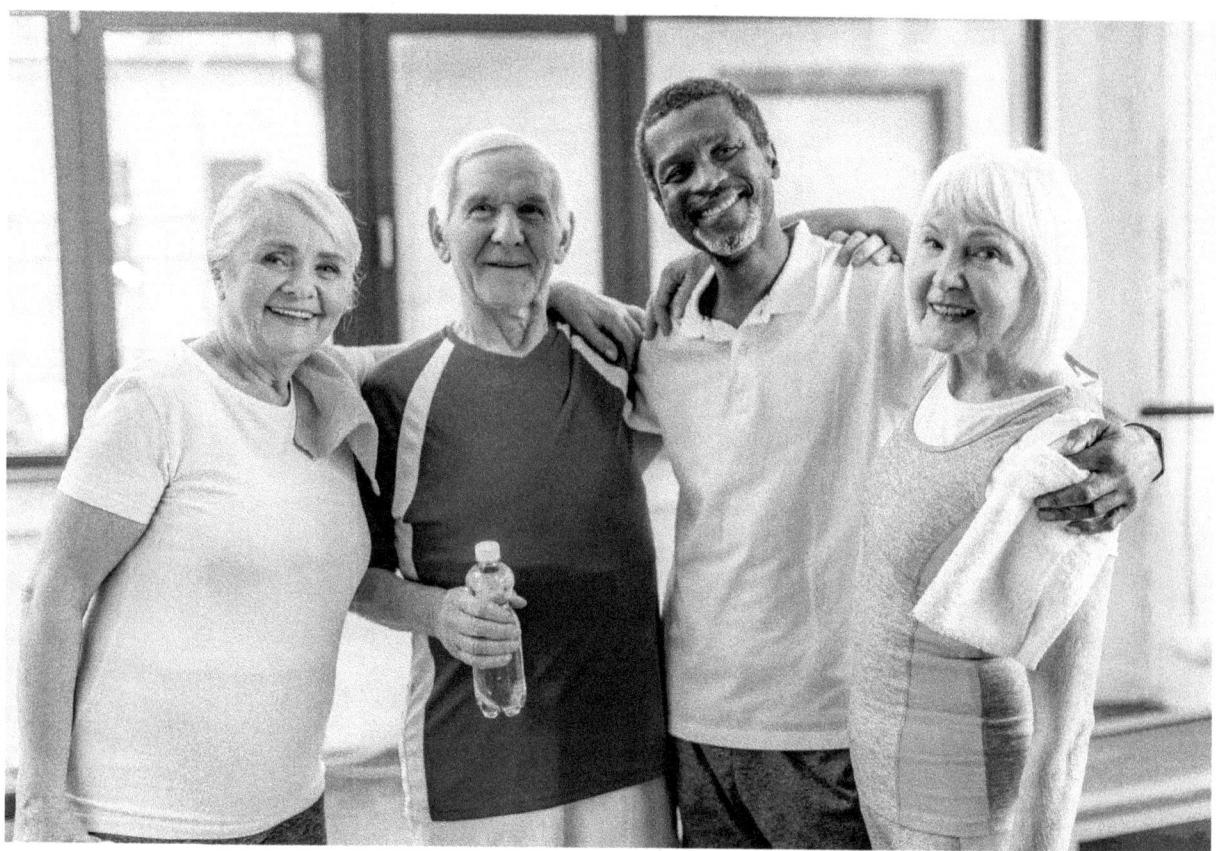

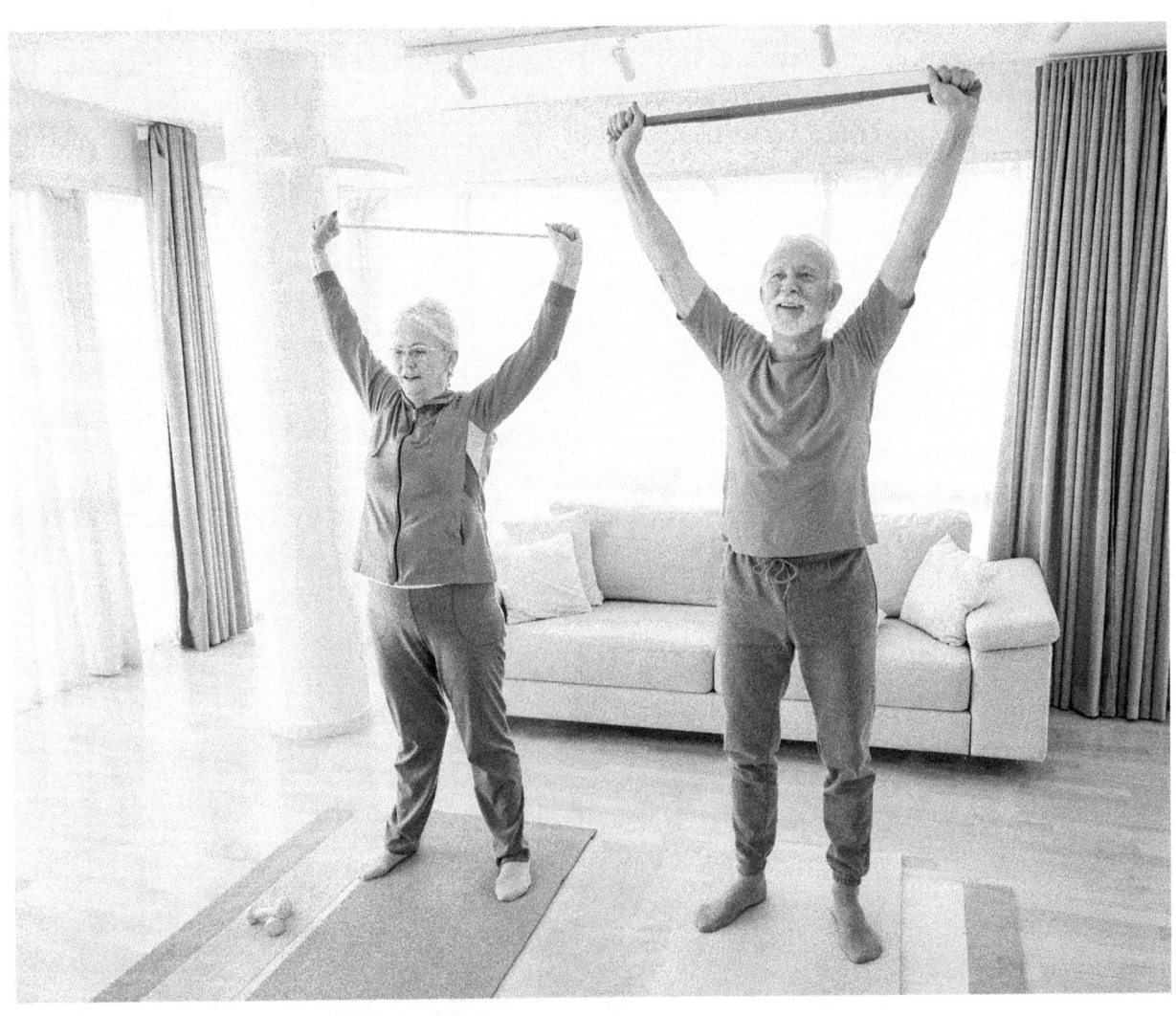

Let's hear it for strength, fitness and weight loss!

CHAPTER 8
Easy Exercises for Strength, Fitness, and Weight Loss

• • • • • • • • • • • •

Now that you've completed the 28-Day Plan, you may want to target specific goals or body areas. That's the purpose of the next few chapters. These are for "do it yourself" exercising where you can customize your own routines; the first being this chapter for Strength, Fitness and Weight Loss. Some exercises cross over to other chapters because they benefit multiple parts of the body. For a more comprehensive workout, continue using the "28-Day Success Plan" with its guided month-long exercises for overall body fitness. You can mix in other exercises from the upcoming targeted routines to change it up a bit. Remember to talk to your doctor before starting any exercise program, including this one. And if you need a visual reference, download the free illustration chart and videos that demonstrate how to perform the exercises in this book. See Chapter 13 for instructions on how to access these.

So, let's get moving with exercises for strength, fitness and weight loss!

Strength, Fitness & Weight Loss

① Tricep/Scapula Stretch

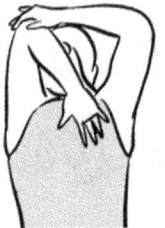

A simple, but very effective stretch that works the Triceps (the backs of your arms above your elbows) and Scapula (the muscles and tissue around and under the shoulder blades). Start facing away from the wall and raise your left arm overhead. Bend your elbow so your arm is behind your head and your hand is on your upper back. Use your right arm to pull your elbow closer to your head and push down slightly. Allow your muscles to gently release as you hold the stretch for 30 seconds. Repeat with the opposite arm.

② The Scoop

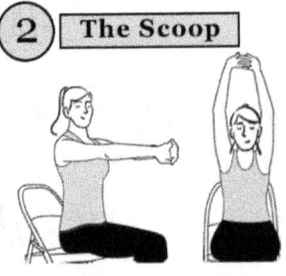

Works the Shoulders, Chest, Spine and Back for flexibility, energy, and better concentration. Begin by interlocking your fingers and inhale as you bring them towards your chin. Exhale slowly as you straighten your elbows and turn your interlocked palms outward, fully extending your arms. Raise your hands above your head with your palms towards the ceiling. Release your hands, turn your palms out, and bring them slowly to your sides. Repeat five times.

③ Cactus Arms

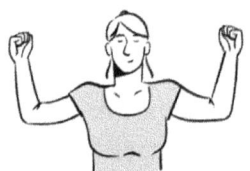 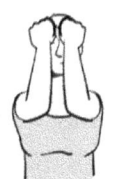

If you're often at a desk or computer, this one's for you! Start with your back and body against the wall. Extend your arms straight out from your sides like an airplane and bend up at the elbow like a cactus. The back of your hands and forearms should be touching the wall. With arms still bent, move them forward so that your palms and forearms come together in front of you. Hold briefly and return to start. Repeat 15 times.

④ Lateral Leg Swings

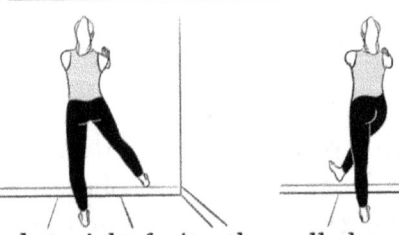

Stand straight facing the wall about three feet away with your palms on the wall. Keeping your legs and knees straight, swing your right leg in front of you towards the left then back over towards the right. Avoid twisting your hips. Do this 5-10 times. Switch legs and repeat on the opposite side and two times each side.

⑤ Bird Flap

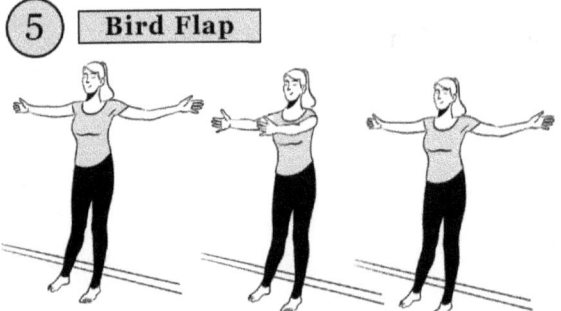

Stand with your back on the wall and feet about two feet asay. Spread your arms straight out as if you're going to hug someone, with the backs of your arms and hands touching the wall and your palms facing out. Keeping your elbows locked, bring your arms straight out in front of you so that your thumbs are up and your palms are facing each other and nearly touching. Hold momentarily and then return your arms to the wall. That's one. Repeat for total of 15-20 reps.

⑥ Large Arm Circles

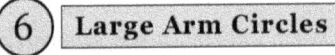

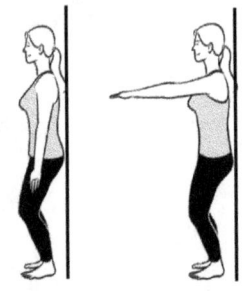 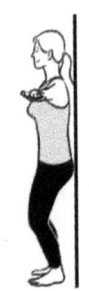 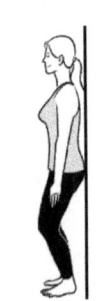

With your back against the wall, bend your knees slightly, raise your arms in front with your elbows locked. Move them out to your sides like an airplane and then down. That's one circle. Do ten slow circles then repeat in the opposite direction. Try varying the size of the circular motion on each set to help work different parts of the muscles.

7) Arms Overhead

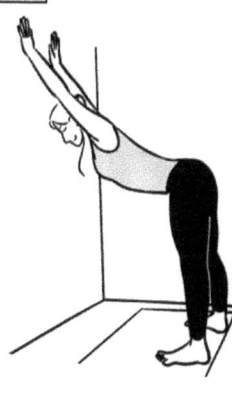

Stand facing the wall, an arm's length away. Raise your arms over your head and place your palms flat against the wall. Keeping your arms straight, lean forward and press your chest towards the wall until you feel a stretch in your upper chest. Hold the stretch for 20-30 seconds, then relax and repeat. For more difficulty, put your palms together as you raise your arms.

8) Standing Knee Extension

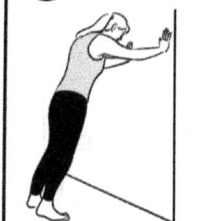 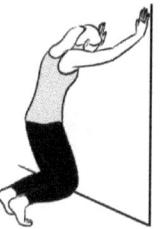 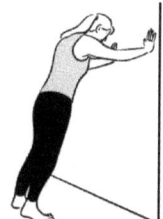

Start by facing the wall about 1 1/2 arm lengths away. Lean over and place your hands on the wall without bending your knees. Keeping your feet in place, slowly bend at the knees towards the wall and hold momentarily before coming back to the starting position. Do this 5-10 times.

9) Side Plank

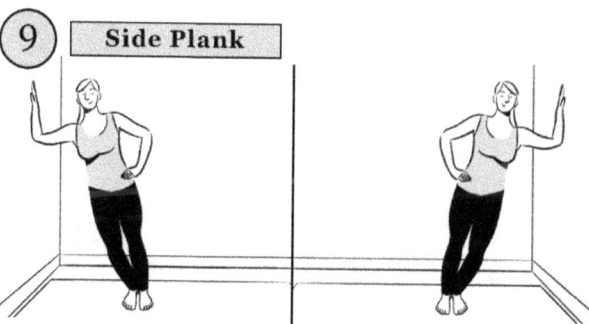

The Side Plank helps with the core and Obliques; the side abdominal muscles that rotate and bend your trunk laterally. Stand next to the wall about three feet away. Put your right hand on your right hip, lean sideways, bend your elbow and place your left forearm on the wall so it's supporting you. Hold for 15 to 30 seconds making sure to keep your body straight. Repeat on the opposite side. That's one set. Do two sets total.

10) Wall Plank

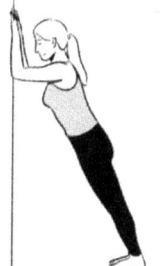 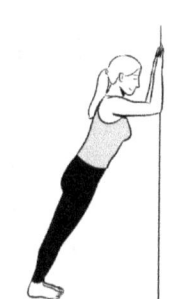

This one works the Abs and Core for strength, stability and balance. Stand facing the wall about one and a half arm's lengths away. Keeping your back straight, lean into the wall, bend your arms and place your forearms and hands on the wall with your palms touching the wall. Hold this position for 30 seconds to two minutes making sure to keep your spine in a straight line. Do not let your hips bend towards the wall!.

11) Hip Circles

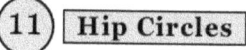
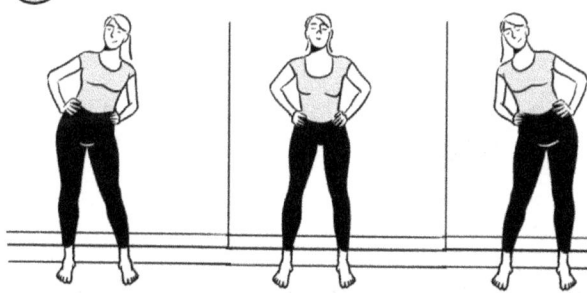

Stand with your back on the wall and feet about two feet asay. Spread your arms straight out as if you're going to hug someone, with the backs of your arms and hands touching the wall and your palms facing out. Keeping your elbows locked, bring your arms straight out in front of you so that your thumbs are up and your palms are facing each other and nearly touching. Hold momentarily and then return your arms to the wall. That's one. Repeat for 15-20 repetitions.

12) Child's Pose

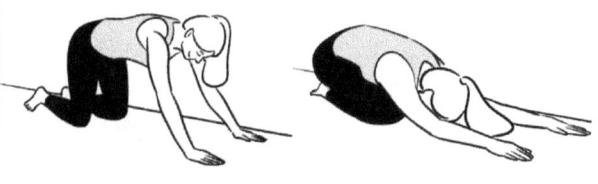

A simple, yet effective, warm-up exercise for the shoulders and to get the blood flowing in the upper body. Also jump starts the your cardio system. Start with your back against the wall, bend your knees slightly, raise your arms in front with your elbows locked. Move them out to your sides like an airplane and then down. That's one circle. Do ten slow circles then repeat the movement in the opposite direction.

13. Tree Pose

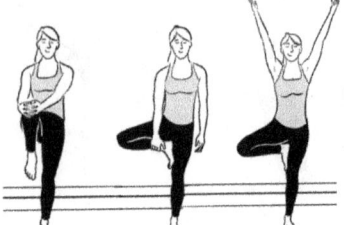

Stand facing away from the wall, close enough for safety. Bend your left knee, grabbing it with your hands and locking them around it. Pause until you are stable and then grab your left foot with your left hand, and bring it up slowly-as high as you can against your right leg with the bottom of your left foot against the side of your right leg. Lock it in if possible then swing your arms up over your head. Hold for 30-60 seconds and then release. Repeat with the opposite leg.

15. Standing Side Lunge

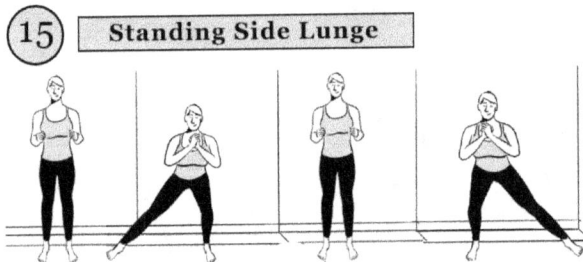

With your back to the wall, Clasp your hands in front of you and bend your elbows. Slide your left foot to the left and bend your left knee while keeping your right leg straight and in place on the floor. Hold momentarily and return to center. Repeat on the opposite side: Slide your right foot to the right and bend your right knee while keeping your left leg straight and in place on the floor. Return to center. That's one. Do 10 total.

17. Wall-Facing Lunge

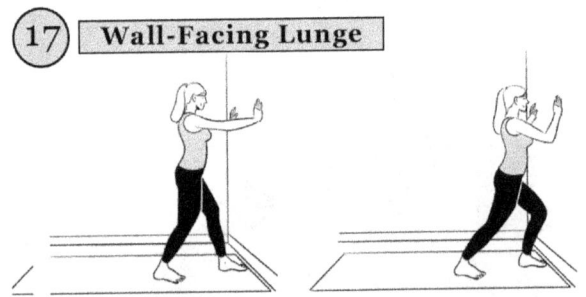

Facing the wall, start by placing your hands on the wall. Step your left foot forward, touching the toes to the wall, while the right foot goes backward. Bend both knees as you bring the left knee close to the wall. The movement should be slow and fluid. Avoid going too low, and keep your shoulders relaxed and your back and shoulders straight. Inhale as you bend your legs forward and exhale as you bring them back. Do a total of 10 repetitions.

14. Tree Pose With Chair

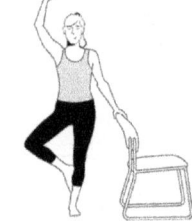

Stand behind the chair with its back to your right and your right hand on the chair for stability. Bend your left knee slowly, bringing your left foot as high as you can against your right leg with the bottom of your foot against the side of your right leg, avoiding the knee area. Lock it in if possible then swing your arms up over your head. If necessary, continue holding the chair for stability. Hold for 30-60 seconds and then release. Repeat with the opposite side.

16. Wall-Supported Lunge

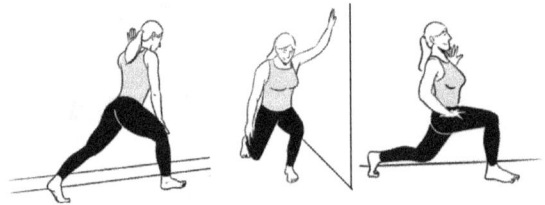

Stand next to the wall an arm's length away looking down the wall. Place your right hand on the wall and your left hand on your hips. Keeping you hips square, bend your left knee as you slide your right leg back behind you into a lunge position, bringing the knee down close to the floor. Hold momentarily, then press the left foot as you pull the right foot back in and squeeze your glutes back to the original position.

18. Mat Wall Bridge

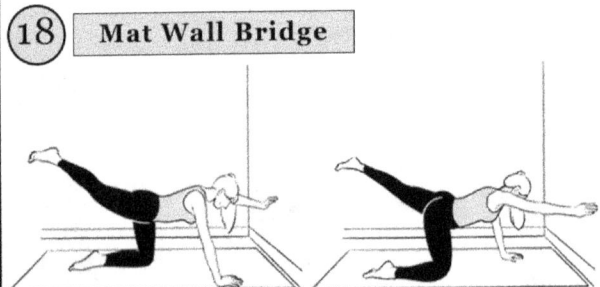

Start facing the wall, about an arm's length away, on your hands and knees. At the same time, reach your left arm out to touch the wall in front of you and your right leg out behind you. Return and repeat with the other side: extend your right arm out to touch the wall and your left leg out behind you. Extend as far as you comfortably can without arching your back. For cardio work, do in quick succession for 10-15 repetitions for each side, pause for 15 seconds and then repeat again.

19) Hip Slides

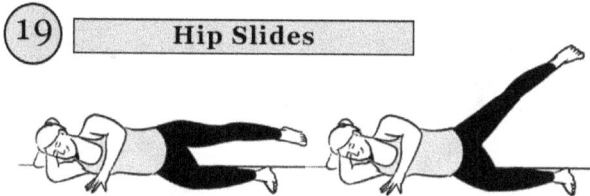

Hip Slides work your core and lower body and are deceptively more difficult than they look. Lie on your side parallel to and facing away from the wall. Both knees should be straight and your top heel should be on the wall. For smoother movement, put a towel between your heel and the wall. Raise your top leg along the wall as high as you can, keeping your heel pressed against the wall. Hold for two seconds then lower. Do this five times then repeat for the opposite side and leg.

20) Wall Teaser

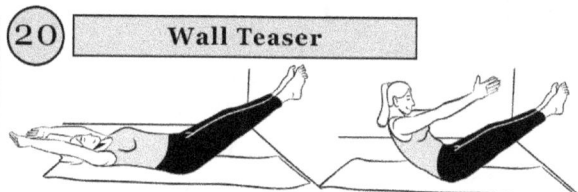

This one mainly works the abs, and is also harder than it looks at first glance. Sit on the floor with your feet on the wall to form a slight "V". Inhale as you slowly roll your body up and move your hands and arms towards your feet until your eyes are level with your toes. Do not jerk the movement up from the floor; make it slow and controlled. Be sure to keep your feet connected to the wall. Hold for a second and then back to the floor. Do 10 times.

21) Balance Bear

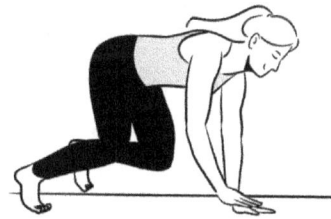

Start on your hands and feet like a bear. Keep your back straight. From this position, lift your right hand and your left foot off the floor an inch or two, then replace. Repeat with other side: lift your left hand and your right foot off the floor an inch or two then replace. That's one repetition. Do a total of five to ten repetitions.

22) Bear Walk Fwd/Back

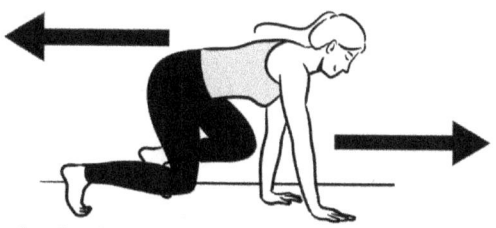

This is the "Balance Bear", but instead of staying in one spot, you actually "walk" across the floor. Start on your hands and feet like a bear. Keep your back straight and slowly walk across the floor in the balance bear stance. Pause, then retrace your steps backwards to your starting spot. Do a total of four repetitions.

23) Bear Walk-Sideways

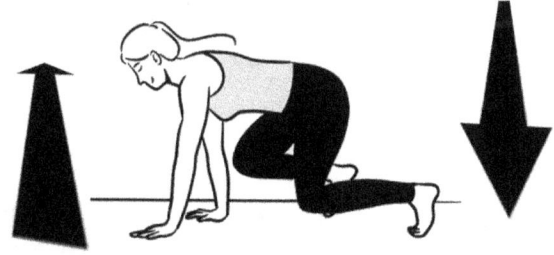

This is the "Bear Walk", but instead of walking straight, you move sideways. Start on your hands and feet like a bear. Keep your back straight and slowly walk sideways in the bear walk stance going first left to right then retracing your steps right to left to your starting position. Do a total of four repetitions.

24) Bear Walk-Circle

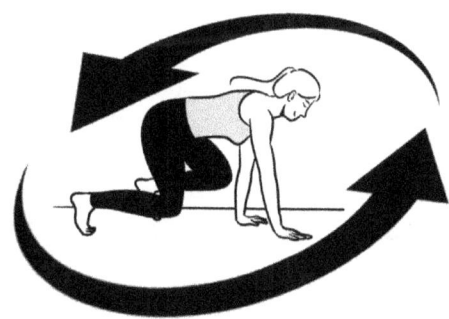

This is the "Bear Walk" but instead of walking straight, you walk in in a circle. Start on your hands and feet like a bear. Keep your back straight and slowly walk clockwise in a circle in the bear walk stance. Do four rotations in each direction. To avoid getting dizzy, move slowly and rest in-between if necessary.

25. Lateral Split Squat

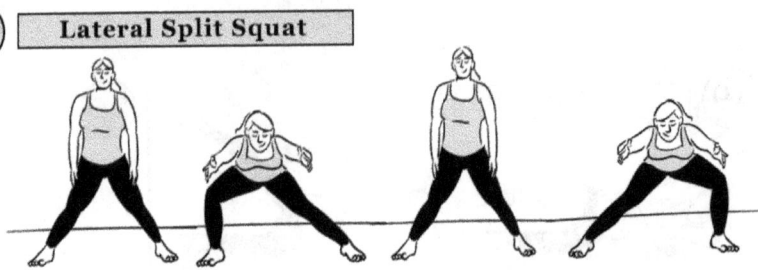

Think of this as a single leg squat to the side. Start with both feet wider than about shoulder distance apart. Lean towards your right leg as you bend your right knee and hip to lower the body. Keep both feet planted on the floor as you continue to lower your body until your right thigh is parallel to the floor. Press downwards with your foot to push your body back up into neutral position. Repeat on the opposite side. That's one. Complete a total of ten repetitions.

26. Side Step

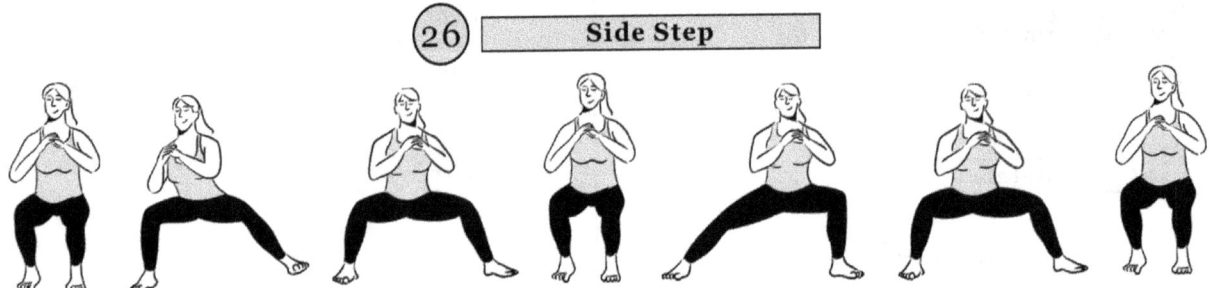

Start in a "wall sit" position with your back against the wall and your knees bent. Bend your elbows and clasp your hands in front of you. Slide your left foot and leg away from your right foot while keeping your body in the same position. Immediately bring your right foot and the rest of your body to the left back towards the other foot and leg so that you are again in a wall squat-your original position. Do this quickly for five steps to the left and then five steps back to the right. Rest momentarily and then repeat in both directions once more.

27. The Frog

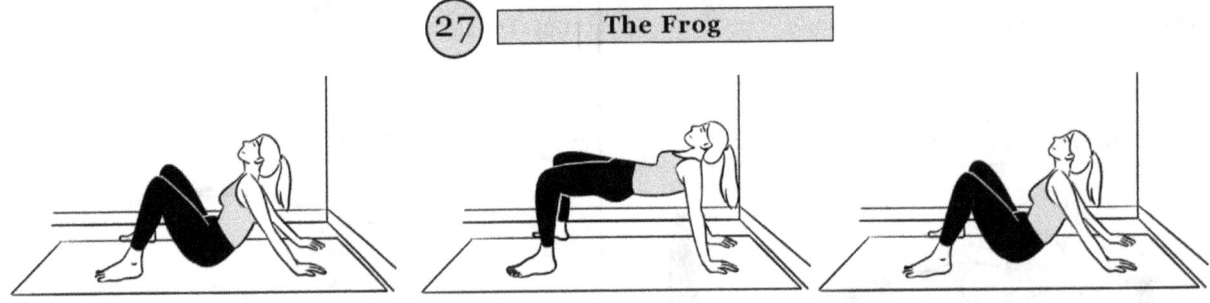

This is a somewhat advanced exercise, so start slow and stretch as much as you can without straining. The more you do the move, the farther you'll be able to stretch. As with all moves, payclose attention to your form and don't overdo it at first. To begin, start in a tabletop or "crab walk" position: with your head, stomach and pelvis pointed towards the ceiling, your feet flat on the floor, knees bent and your hands behind you with your palms on the floor. Keep your arms fully extended and not bent. From here, push your buttocks up to straighten your back and stretch your spine as much as possible. Hold momentarily then return to the starting position. Do this five to ten times.

As you come to the end of these exercises for strength, fitness and weight loss, remember that consistency is the key to your progress. It's not about going hard for a week and then ghosting your mat for a month. It's about showing up day after day, with enthusiasm and anticipation. You can do this!

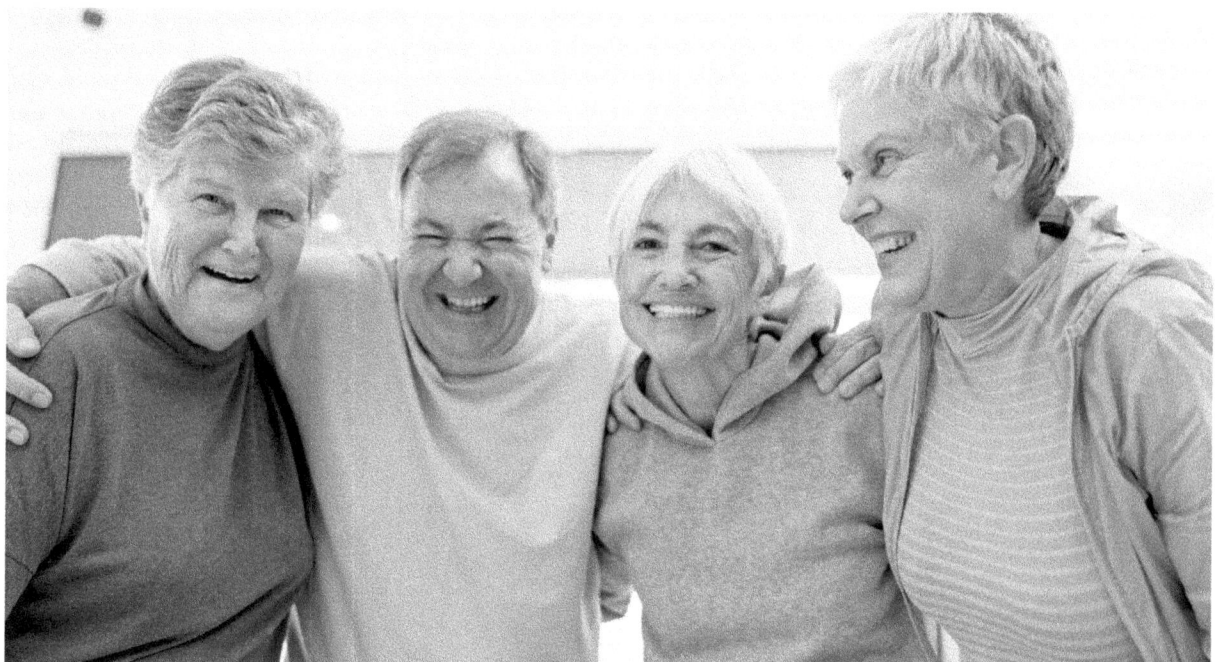

Chapter 9
Targeted Upper Body Exercises

As the years go by, simple tasks can become a real struggle, but upper body exercises can help improve some everyday tasks. By building up those shoulder, arm, and back muscles, we can get through daily activities easier, helping to reduce the risk of strain and injury along the way. A strong upper body isn't just about physical strength – it's also a key to better posture, balance and everyday functioning.

As with the previous chapter, these are for "do it yourself" exercising where you can customize your own routines; this chapter focuses on the upper body, although some exercises cross over from other chapters because they benefit multiple areas. Pick five or six exercises from this group to do as one routine for targeting the upper body. Rotate exercises in and out from the group each time you do a targeted routine. Feel free to add in breathing and stretching exercises from earlier chapters and always talk to your doctor before starting any exercise program, including this one.

Let's get moving with exercises targeting the upper body!

Upper Body Exercises

1. Triceps/Scapula Stretch

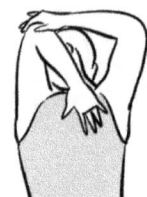

Raise your left arm overhead and bend your elbow so your arm is behind your head and you hand on your upper back. Use your right arm to pull the elbow closer to your head and push down slightly. Hold the stretch for 30 seconds. Repeat with the opposite arm for a total of twice each side.

2. The Scoop

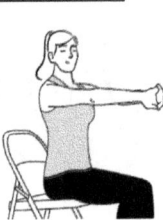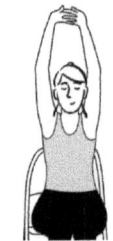

With your arms down, interlock your fingers with palms facing up. Inhale deeply as you bring your palms towards your chin. Turn your palms outward and exhale as you straighten your elbows until your arms are fully extended in front of you. Keep the motion going as you raise your interlocked hands above your head with your palms towards the ceiling. Hold momentarily, then release your hands to bring them to your sides. Do five reps.

3. Bent Arm Pec Stretch

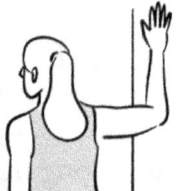

Find a wall where the corner juts out. Stand parallel to the wall with the corner behind you. Bend your left arm at the elbow and place your upper forearm and palm on the parallel wall behind you. Rotate your body to the right to feel the stretch. Hold 5-10 seconds then repeat with the other arm.

4. Standing Wall Stretch

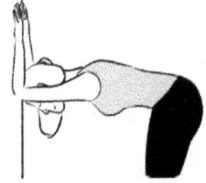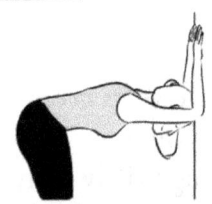

Stand about half an arm's length away and facing the wall. Keeping your legs straight, bend at the waist, put your elbows and forearms on the wall as you breathe out. Hold for 10 seconds. Relax and repeat. Be mindful of your breathing while performing the stretch.

5. Arm Raises Against Wall

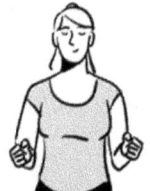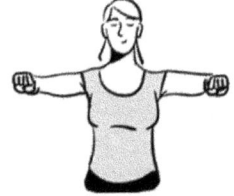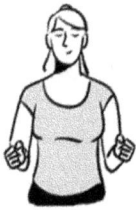

Stand upright with your back against the wall so that your head, buttocks, and upper back are firmly pressed against it. Your feet should not be too far apart. Bend your elbows to form a 90° angle. Raise your arms and begin the movement, sliding your elbows along your sides. Keep your arms and back against the wall at all times. Inhale when raising your arms and exhale when returning to the starting position. To make it easier, you can slightly bend your knees so that your back adheres even more to the wall.

6. Cactus Arms

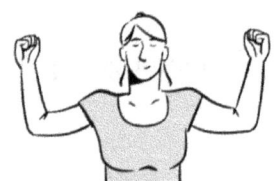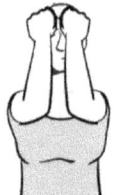

Start with your back and body against the wall and your arms bent up at the elbow at a 90-degree angle like a cactus. The important part of this stretch is to get the back of your hands and forearms to touch the wall. Move your arms forward so that your palms and forearms come together in front of you. Pause briefly. With elbows still bent, then move your arms back so your forearms and outer hands touch the wall. Hold for three seconds. Repeat 10 times.

7. Wall Angels

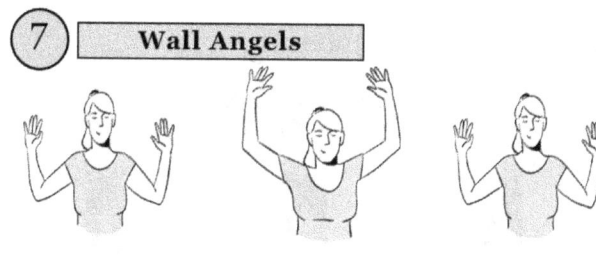

Stand with your back to the wall and feet about six inches away. Bend your arms 90 degrees while keeping them as flat against the wall as possible. From that position, keep your back and arms on the wall and slowly raise your arms up as far as possible. Hold briefly at the top and bring back down to the starting position. Repeat five times. Be sure to keep your arms pressed against the wall as much as you can at all times.

8. Cat-Cow

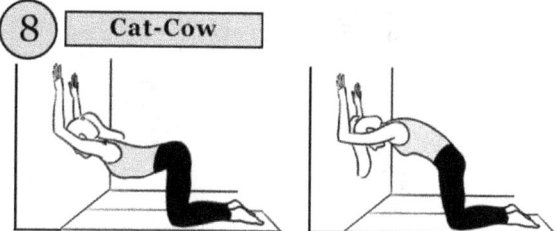

Get on your hands and knees facing the wall about an arm's length away. Lean into the wall and put your elbows, forearms and palms on the wall while arching your back. Hold for three seconds while inhaling and exhaling, then roll your back down while sticking your buttocks out. your back should now be in a simi "U" shape. Hold for five seconds while you inhale and exhale then return.

9. Reach-Twist-Wrap

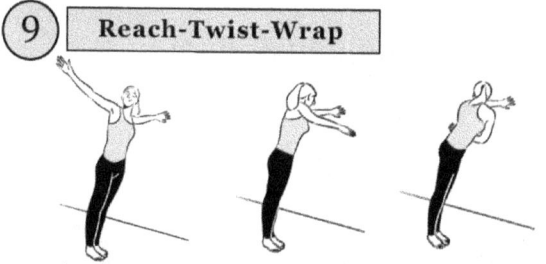

Stand an arm's length away from wall, facing parallel to it. Bend your left arm, lean your body and place your forearm against the wall while keeping your side straight. Reach your right arm out to your side and slightly up and hold briefly as you inhale. Exhale and twist your body to the left while bringing your right arm down and under the left arm while keeping it extended and away from you to "wrap" your body. Do 3-5 times each side.

10. Kneeling Archer

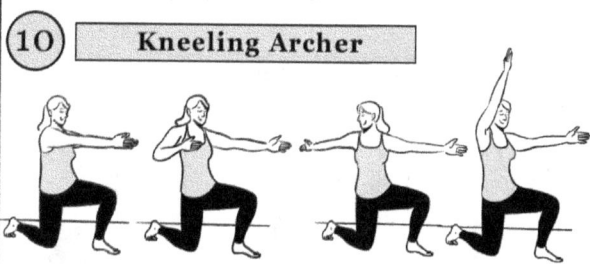

Start by kneeling down on your right knee and your right leg bent so your foot is flat on the floor. Extend your arms in front of you with your palms together. Keep your left arm still as you pull your right arm straight back and rotate your torso while extending your right arm behind you and, in a circular motion, raise your right arm over your head and down in front of you to join the other palm. Repeat three times with each side.

11. Bird Flap

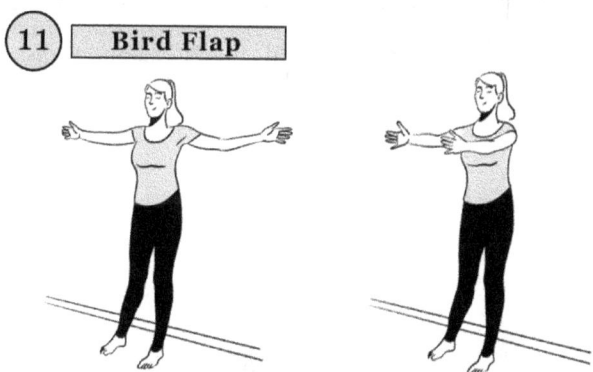

Stand with you back to the wall, glutes and shoulders touching. Your feet should be about two feet away. Spread your arms straight out like an airplane, with the backs of your arms and hands touching the wall and your palms facing out. Keeping your elbows locked, bring your arms straight out in front of you so that your thumbs are up and your palms are facing each other and nearly touching. Hold momentarily and then return your arms to the wall. That's one. Repeat at a medium speed 15 times. Rest 30 seconds, then repeat.

12. Arms Overhead

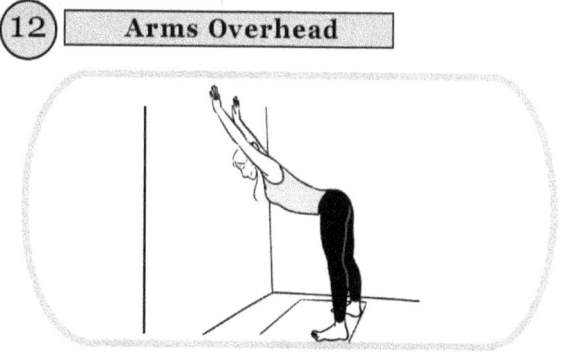

Stand facing the wall, an arm's length away. Raise your arms over your head and place your palms flat against the wall. Keeping your arms straight, lean forward and press your chest towards the wall until you feel a stretch in your upper chest and back. Hold the stretch for 20-30 seconds, then relax and repeat. For more difficulty, put your palms together as you raise your arms. you can also perform this exercise by placing your hands on the counter or a chair back instead of the wall, which will allow you to bend lower.

13. Side Bend/Side Stretch

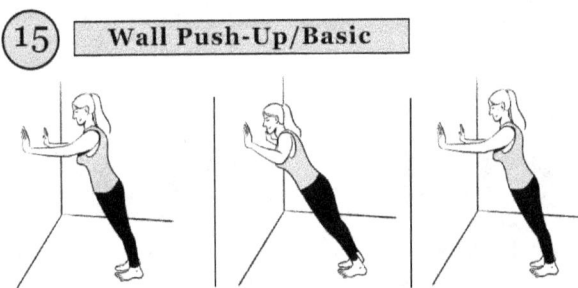

Stand sideways next to the wall, with your right side closest to the wall and feet hip-width apart. Extend your left arm overhead, placing your right hand on the wall for support. Gently slide your right hand down the wall as you bend your torso to the right, feeling a stretch along the left side of your body. Hold the stretch for 20-30 seconds, then repeat with the opposite side for three sets.

14. Lateral Raises

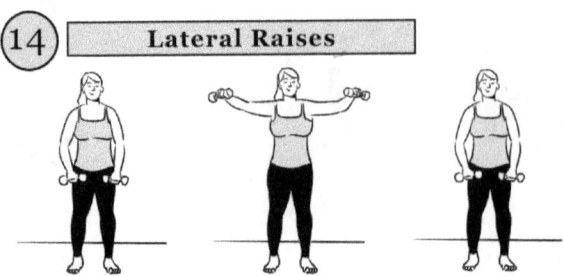

This exercise can use weights or not, depending on your level. Stand upright with your arms bent at the elbows. Bring both elbows straight up to shoulder level as if pouring water out of a pitcher. Bring back to start and repeat. Do this 6-10 times. Increase weight as you get stronger.

15. Wall Push-Up/Basic

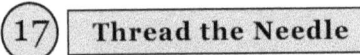

Stand about an arms' length from a wall. Place your palms flat on the wall, slightly wider than shoulder-width apart, with your arms straight, and your fingers pointing upward. Take a small step back, so you are leaning against your hands. Keeping your spine straight, slowly bend your arms until your head touches the wall. Pause. Slowly push yourself away from the wall and back up. That's one. Do this 10-15 times.

16. Multi-Stretch

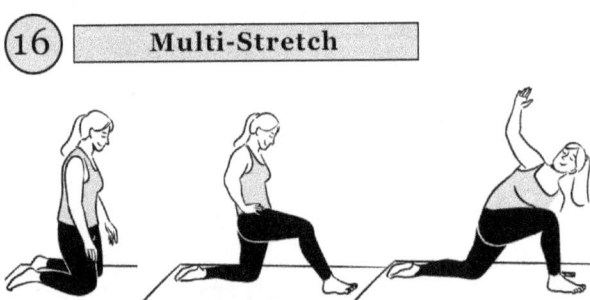

Start on your knees parallel to the wall. Stretch your left leg out in front of you with your leg bent and the foot flat on the floor. Lean forward with your torso to add a stretch to the planted knee's hip flexor. Place one hand on the floor opposite to the front foot. Finally, reach your left arm up and rotate towards the ceiling leading with your upper back and shoulders. Hold for 3 seconds then repeat on the opposite side.

17. Thread the Needle

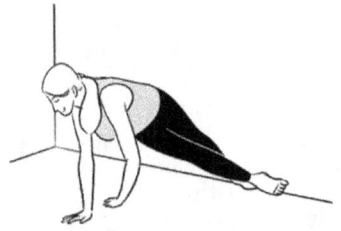

Start on your belly in the push-up position. Place your feet in the crevice between the wall and floor with your left toes touching your right heel. Lift your left arm to the ceiling and then rotate your torso to bring your left arm slowly back down between your chest and the floor. Repeat five times then switch sides.

18. Child's Pose

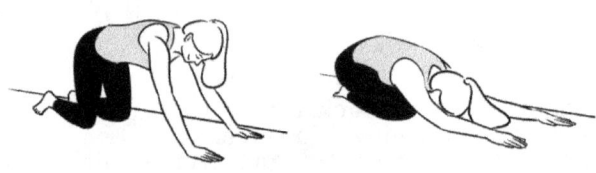

Start on hands and knees with your arms stretched out slightly in front of you. Bend back, bending your knees and folding your upper body so that you are almost sitting on your legs. Stretch out your arms with your palms on the floor. Hold for 20 seconds and repeat three times.

We've come to the end of our exercises targeting the upper body.

These exercises are tools for preserving independence and enhancing our quality of life. Our goal is to gain functional strength that supports our lifestyles and passions. For a more comprehensive workout, continue using the "28-Day Success Plan" with its guided month-long exercises for overall body fitness to help get you moving and keep you active every day of the week.

If you haven't done so yet, be sure to download the free Wall Pilates reference chart. We also have free demonstration videos showing how to properly do the exercises in this book. See Chapter 13 for instructions on how to access these.

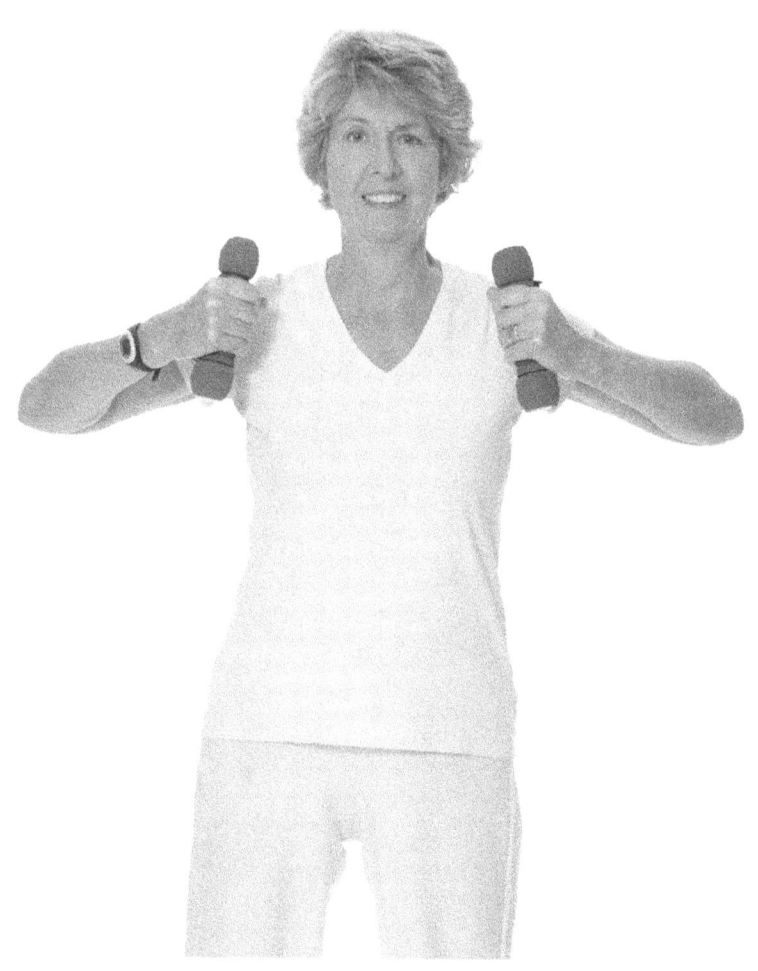

Chapter 10
Exercises for Balance & Coordination

• • • ● • ● • ● • •

Balance and coordination can become key issues as we get older. This can happen for a number of reasons, but many times, it's because some key muscles are getting weaker and smaller, which makes it harder for our body to stay steady when we move. In addition, our senses change. We might not be able to feel where our body is in "space" as well as we used to, and the part of our inner ear that helps us stay balanced might not work as well. This can make us feel dizzy or wobbly.

While we can't fix issues related to medical problems, there are things we can do to help steady ourselves as we age, including exercises that focus on the primary muscles that aid our balance and coordination and that's what this chapter is all about. Pick five or six exercises from this group to do as one routine for targeting balance and coordination. Rotate exercises in and out from the group each time you do this targeted routine. And please talk to your doctor before starting any exercise program, including this one.

Exercises for Balance & Coordination

1. Triceps/Scapula Stretch

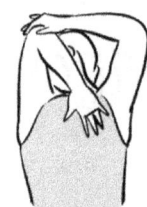

Raise your left arm overhead and bend your elbow so your arm is behind your head and you hand on your upper back. Use your right arm to pull the elbow closer to your head and push down slightly. Hold the stretch for 30 seconds. Repeat with the opposite arm for a total of twice each side.

2. Single Arm Pec Stretch

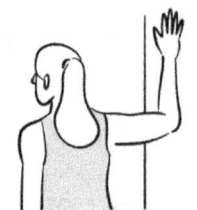 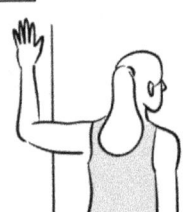

Find a wall where the corner juts out. Stand parallel to the wall with the corner behind you. Bend your left arm at the elbow and place your upper forearm and palm on the parallel wall behind you. Rotate your body to the right to feel the stretch. Hold 5-10 seconds then repeat with the other arm.

3. The Scoop

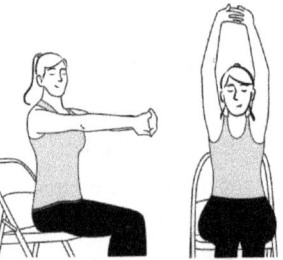

With your arms down, interlock your fingers with palms facing up. Inhale deeply as you bring your palms towards your chin.

Turn your palms outward and exhale slowly as you straigh as you straighten your elbows until your arms are fully extended in front of you. Keep the motion going as you raise your interlocked hands above your head with your palms towards the ceiling. Hold momentarily, then release your hands to bring them to your sides. Do five slow repetitions, concentrating on form and breathing.

4. Arms Overhead

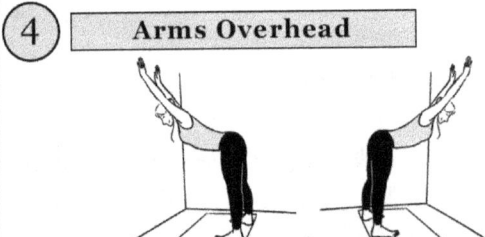

Stand facing the wall, an arm's length away. Raise your arms over your head and place your palms flat against the wall. Keeping your arms straight, lean forward and press your chest towards the wall until you feel a stretch in your upper chest. Hold the stretch for 20-30 seconds, then relax and repeat. For more difficulty, put your palms together as you raise your arms.

5. Bird Flap

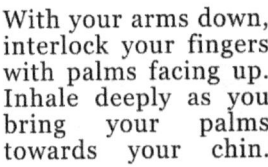

Stand with you back to the wall, glutes and shoulders touching. Your feet should be about two feet away. Spread your arms straight out like an airplane, with the backs of your arms and hands touching the wall and your palms facing out. Keeping your elbows locked, bring your arms straight out in front of you so that your thumbs are up and your palms are facing each other and nearly touching. Hold briefly and then return your arms to the wall. That's one. Repeat at a medium speed 15 times.

6. Large Hip Circles

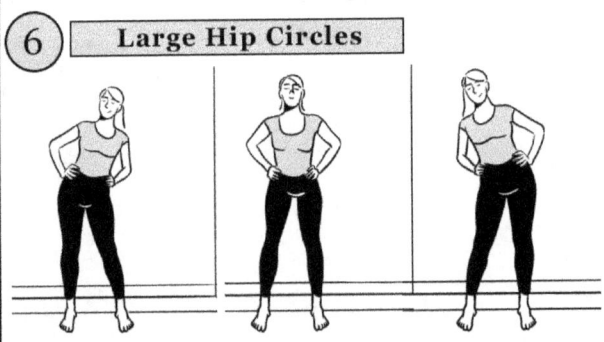

Stand facing away from the wall, with your feet spread shoulder-width apart about three feet from the wall. Put your hands on your hips and pull your stomach in so that you engage your core muscles. Bend to the side slightly as you and rotate your hips clockwise 10 times at a medium speed. Repeat in the opposite direction 10 more times. Gradually increase the size of the circles as you become more flexible and comfortable with the exercise.

7. Hip Flexor Stretch

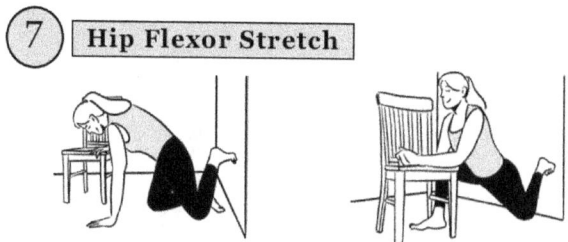

With a chair sideways in front of you, kneel down with your back to and your feet touching the wall. Lean forward so your right hand is on the chair and your left hand is on the floor. Put your left foot on the wall with the ball of your foot touching. Bring your right foot forward and bend your knee so your foot is flat on the floor. Put your right hand on the floor and push your pelvis forward and away from the wall to feel the stretch. Hold for 3-5 seconds. Unwind and repeat with the opposite leg on the wall.

8. Flamingo

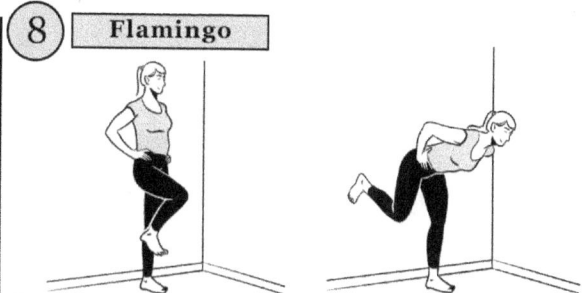

Stand on your left foot and bend your right knee so your right foot is next to your left knee and pointed straight out. Place your hands on your hips and find your balance. Hinge forward, extending your right leg backward and upward to touch the wall behind you. Return to the start. Do five reps on the right side, then switch to having the left up while standing on your right foot.

9. Flying Flamingo

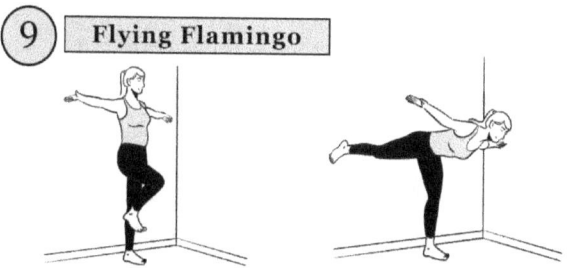

Same as the Flamingo, but with arms extended like an airplane and your back leg extended straight. Stand on your left foot and bend your right knee so your right foot is next to your left knee and pointed straight out. Put your hands on your hips to balance. Extend your arms out like an airplane and hinge forward, moving your right leg rearward and upward. Return to the start. Do five reps on the right side, then switch to having the left foot up while standing on your right leg.

10. Standing Bicycle

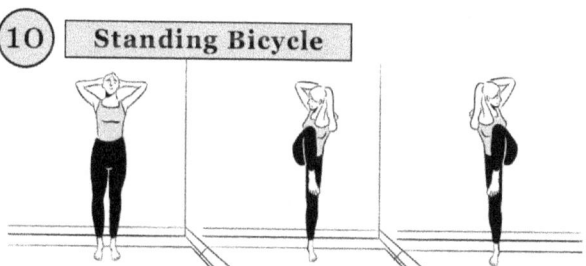

Lean your back and glutes against the wall and put your hands behind your head with your feet close together. Lift your right knee and left elbow simultaneously, trying to touch or get them as close together as possible. Perform the same movement with your left knee and right elbow. Alternate as quickly as possible between right and left sides while trying not to lift your back off the wall. Inhale with your feet on the floor and exhale as you bring your knee toward your elbow.

11. Lateral Leg Swing

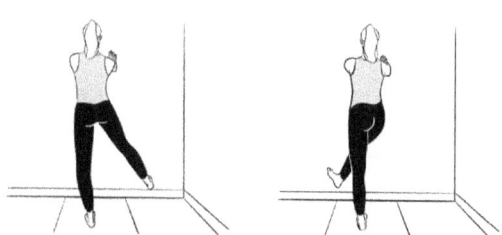

Lean in from a bit more than an arm's length away and place your palms on the wall. From this position, exhale and swing your right leg laterally in front of your left leg towards your left side. Inhale as you return. Do this ten times then repeat with the left leg. Exhale as you swing it laterally in front of your right leg and towards your right side. Inhale as you return. Keep your legs and knees straight, and avoid twisting your hips. Do two or three total sets.

12. Side Leg Lifts

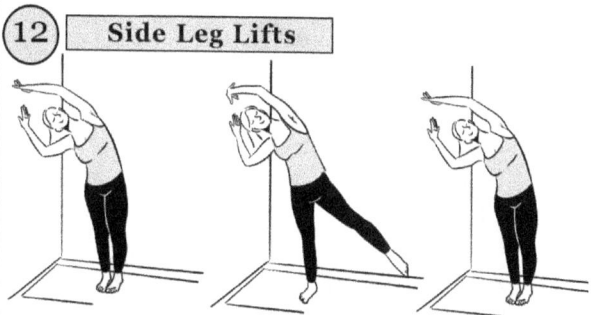

Begin by standing sideways arm's length from the wall, with your right side closest to the wall and feet hip-width apart. Put your right forearm on the wall, extend your left arm overhead, and slide your right hand down the wall as you bend your torso to the right. Hold this position for 5-10 seconds to allow your obliques to stretch. Next, lift your left leg up and out sideways for ten repetitions. Switch sides and repeat the entire process.

13. Reverse (Rear) leg Lifts

Start by facing the wall a bit more than an arm's length away. Bend at the waist keeping your body straight and put your palms on the wall bending until your body forms an "L". Keeping your hips pointing towards the floor, swing your right leg out behind you and up as far as you comfortably can. Hold for 1 second and bring back to the start position. That's one. Repeat for a total of ten repetitions then switch to the left leg for ten reps.

14. Reverse Lunge

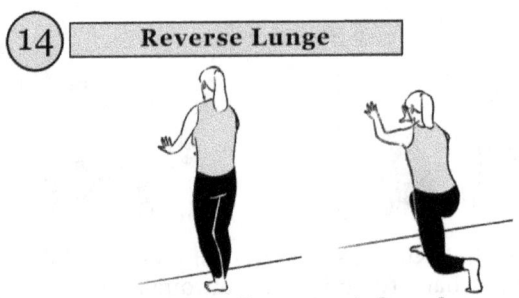

Stand facing the wall, an arm's length away, and your feet a few inches apart. Place your hands against the wall, bend your right knee as you step backwards with your left leg into a lunge. Go as far back as possible with your right knee never going beyond the toes. Return to the starting position, and repeat on the opposite side. Do this five times on each side.

15. Press Lunge

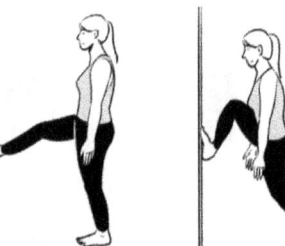

Begin by standing one leg-length away from the wall. Find your balance and then place your right foot on the wall at hip-height, leaving your left leg straight. Bend your right knee and lunge forward until your knee is pointed up, keeping your upper body neutral and upright. Pause for one second, then press forcefully through the ball of your foot to return to your starting position. Repeat ten times then switch sides. For a more difficult workout, alternate legs between reps.

16. Wall Sit

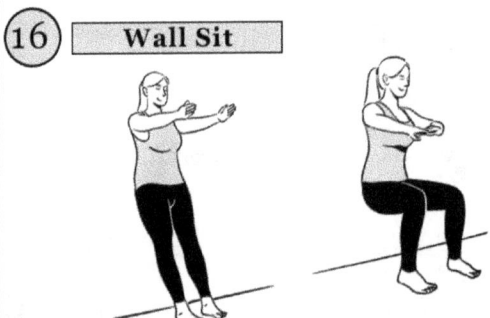

Stand with your back against the wall and your feet shoulder-width apart. walk your feet out slightly so that your back is leaning against the wall slightly. Slowly lower your body down the wall, keeping your feet flat on the floor. Stop when your thighs are parallel to the floor. If you can't see your toes, your feet are too far in towards the wall. Hold for 60 seconds. Repeat.

17. Wall Sit/Leg Out

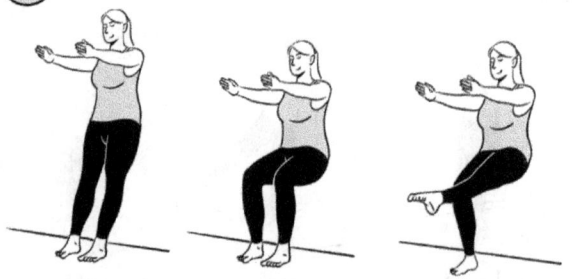

Stand with your back on the wall and your feet shoulder-width apart. Hold your hands out in front of you for balance. Bend your knees, lowering your hips deeply so your thighs are parallel with the floor, keeping weight back in your heels. Slowly raise your right leg out so that it is straight with your toes pointed. Hold for 30 seconds. Rise back up and repeat the motion, this time raising the right leg. Relax.

18. Split Squat

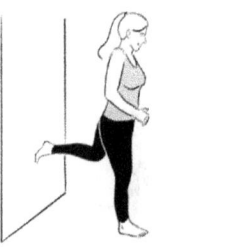 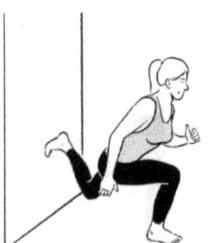

Stand facing away from the wall about three feet away. Bend your left knee and place your left foot on the wall behind you. Using your arms to balance you, bend down into a squatting position while keeping your left foot on the wall. Immediately return to the starting position. Quickly do 8-10 repetitions and then switch legs. You can also alternate legs between repetitions if desired.

19) Single Leg Squat

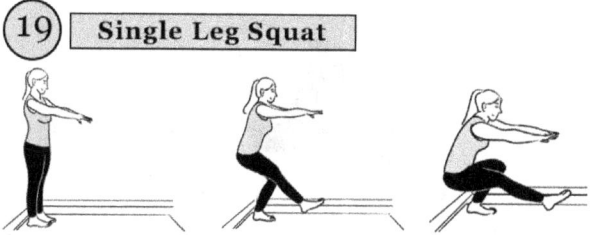

Start with your back on the wall and our feet about one foot from it and arms at your side. Bend your right leg to lift your foot off the ground slightly so that your weight is on your left foot. Bend your left knee as you squat down, keeping your left foot flat on the floor and your right foot elevated. Stop and hold before your leg is parallel to the floor. Push back up and repeat five times. Switch and repeat with the right leg bearing your weight.

20) Squat with Calf Raise

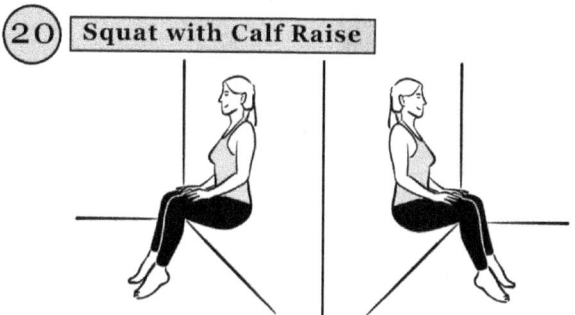

Begin in a wall squat with your back on the wall and your legs bent so your thighs are parallel with the floor. Next, lift your heels off the ground. Hold briefly then return your heel to the floor, and push up out of the squat. Repeat 5-10 times.

21) Squat with Cactus Arms

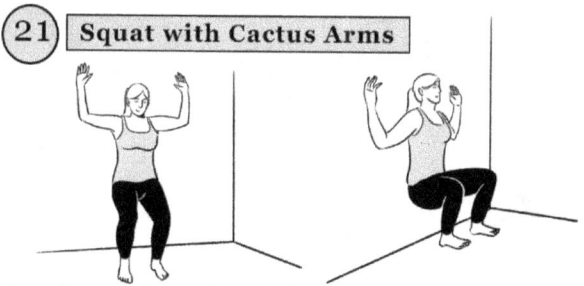

Stand straight and upright with your arms out like an airplane and your back against the wall. Bend your elbows so that your hands are pointing up while walking your feet out in front slightly. Slide down into a squat by bending your knees until thighs are parallel with the floor. Keep arms out or bring your elbows in so that they nearly touch each other. Hold momentarily and then push back up while bringing your elbows back out to the original position. Repeat for 5-10 repetitions.

22) Forward Squat

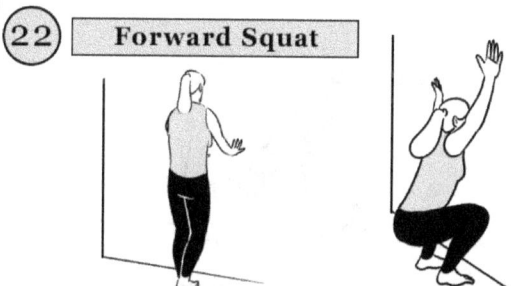

Start facing the wall with your feet shoulder length apart and your toes about a foot from the wall. Keeping you head up, lift your arms above your head and squat down until your thighs are parallel with the floor. Hold for a second, push back up. Repeat 8-10 times. As you get more comfortable, put your feet closer to the wall, but make sure to keep your back straight and your head up.

23) Wall Tree Pose

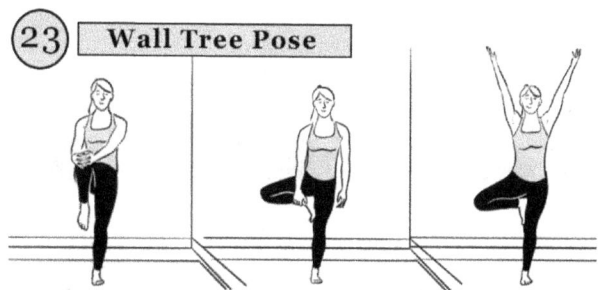

For beginners, use the wall for balance. Stand facing away from the wall slightly and bend your right knee, grabbing it with your hands and locking them around it. Pause until you are stable and then grab your right foot with your right hand, twisting it slightly so that the inner thigh is looking upward. Bring it up slowly-as high as you can against your left leg with the bottom of your right foot against the side of your left leg. Lock it in if possible then swing your arms up over your head. Hold for 30-60 seconds and then release. Repeat with left leg.

24) Tree with Chair

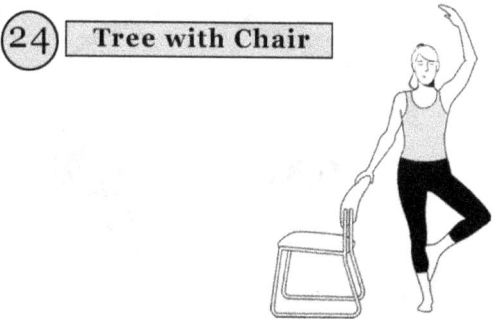

Great for beginners and those with balance challenges. Stand behind the chair with its back to your right and your right hand on the chair for stability. Bend your left knee slowly, bringing your left foot as high as you can against your right leg with the bottom of your foot against the side of your right leg, avoiding the knee area. Lock it in if possible then swing your arms up over your head. If necessary, continue holding the chair for stability. Hold for 30-60 seconds and then release. Repeat with the opposite side.

25. Balance Bear

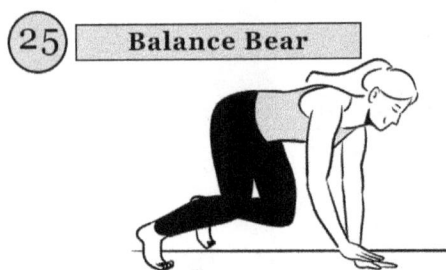

Start on your hands and feet like a bear. Keep your back straight. From this position, lift your right hand and your left foot off the floor an inch or two, then replace. Repeat with other side: lift your left hand and your right foot off the floor an inch or two then replace. That's one repetition. Do a total of five to ten repetitions.

26. Bear Walk-Forwards

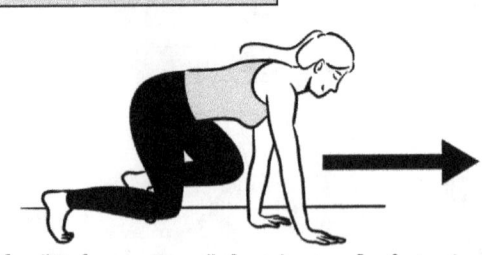

This is the "Balance Bear", but instead of staying in one spot, you actually "walk" across the floor. Start on your hands and feet like a bear. Keep your back straight and slowly walk across the floor in the balance bear stance. Pause, then retrace your steps backwards to your starting spot. Do a total of four repetitions.

27. Bear Walk-Backwards

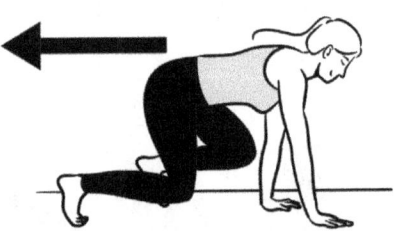

This is the "Balance Bear", but instead of staying in one spot, you actually "walk" across the floor. Start on your hands and feet like a bear. Keep your back straight and slowly walk across the floor in the balance bear stance. Pause, then retrace your steps backwards to your starting spot. Do a total of four repetitions.

28. Bear Walk-Sideways

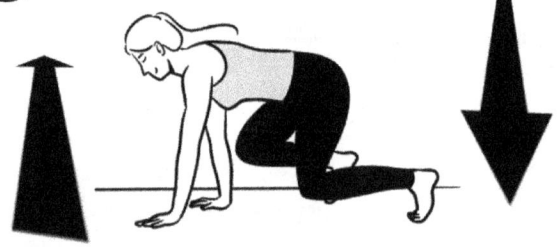

This is the "Bear Walk", but instead of walking straight, you move sideways. Start on your hands and feet like a bear. Keep your back straight and slowly walk sideways in the bear walk stance going first left to right then retracing your steps right to left to your starting position. Do a total of four repetitions.

29. Bear Walk-Circle

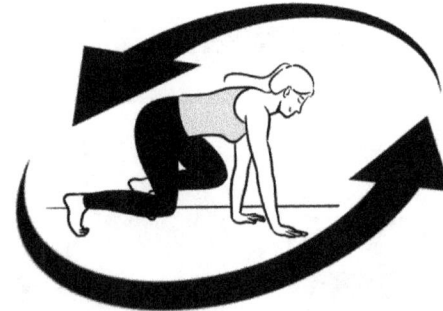

This is the "Bear Walk" but instead of walking straight, you walk in in a circle. Start on your hands and feet like a bear. Keep your back straight and slowly walk clockwise in a circle in the bear walk stance. Do four rotations in each direction. To avoid getting dizzy, move slowly and rest in-between if necessary.

30. Half Windmill Sit

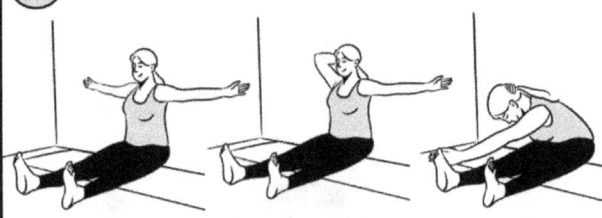

Sit on the floor with your back to the wall and your arms straight out like an airplane with your palms facing out. Bend your elbow to place your right hand on the back of your head. Swing your left arm around to the outside of your RIGHT knee and keeping your back straight, bend to put the back of your left hand on the outside of your right foot. Hold for five seconds then back to the neutral position. Repeat on the opposite side and five times total.

That's it for this chapter focusing on balance and coordination. For a more complete workout, continue using the "28-Day Success Plan" with its guided month-long exercises for overall body fitness to help get you moving and keep you active every day of the week. Use selected exercises from these targeted routines to personalize that plan and make it your own.

If you haven't done so yet, be sure to download the free Wall Pilates reference chart. We also have free demonstration videos showing how to properly do the exercises in this book. See Chapter 13 for instructions on how to access these.

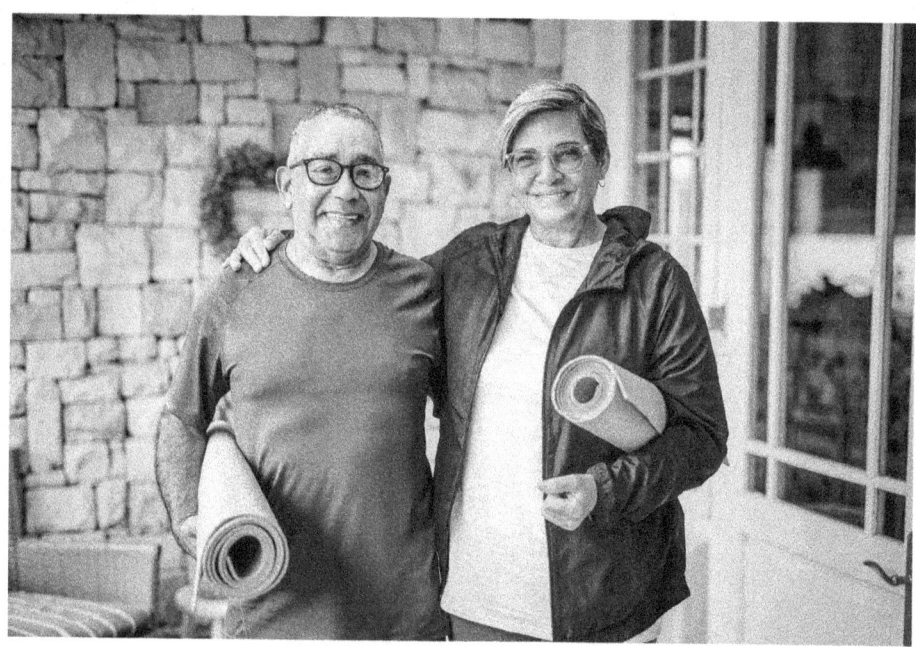

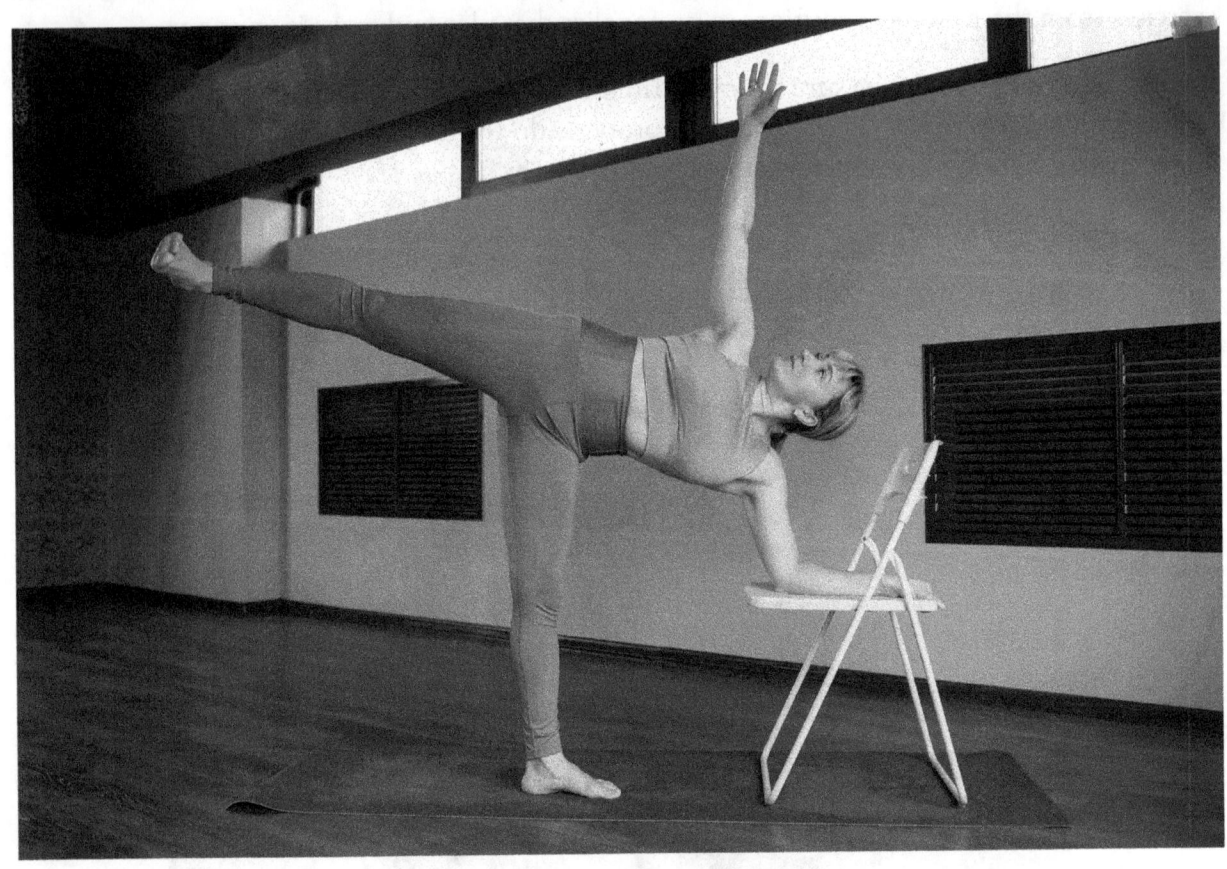

Let's strengthen that lower body!

Chapter 11
Lower-Body Exercises

• • • ● • ● • ● • • •

There are things we can do to help steady ourselves as we age. Like following a regular exercise regimen that focuses on muscles that help us walk, bend and move; and that's what this chapter is all about. Strengthening your thighs, quads, hips and calves isn't just about building muscle. It's also about getting around; keeping your mobility and independence through functional fitness. And we don't just focus on isolated muscle groups; we're using exercises that mimic real-life movements and everyday tasks like climbing stairs or bending down to pet the cat.

Pick five or six exercises from this group to do as a routine for targeting balance and coordination. Rotate exercises in and out from the group each time you do a targeted routine.

As with the previous four chapters, this one is also for "do it yourself" exercising where you can customize the routines to fit your level and style. Some exercises cross over from other chapters due to their benefits to multiple parts of the body. For a more rounded workout with specific day-by-day exercises, continue with the "28-Day Success Plan" in chapters 6 and 7. The plan's step-by-step exercises work together for overall body fitness packaged into a month-long guided program. And be sure to talk to your doctor before starting any exercise program, including this one.

Let's get started with some traditional warm-ups.

Lower-Body Exercises

1. Lateral Leg Swings

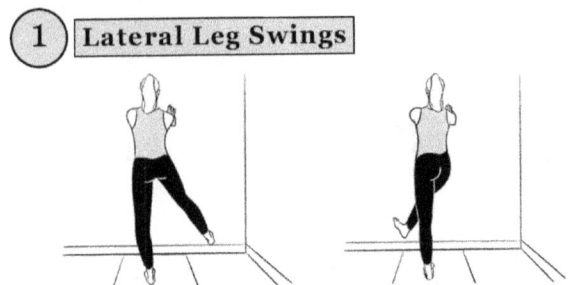

Stand straight facing the wall about three feet away with your palms on the wall. Keeping your legs and knees straight, swing your right leg in front of you towards the left then back over towards the right. Avoid twisting your hips. Do this 5-10 times. Switch legs and repeat on the opposite side and two times each side.

2. Reverse (Rear) Leg Lifts

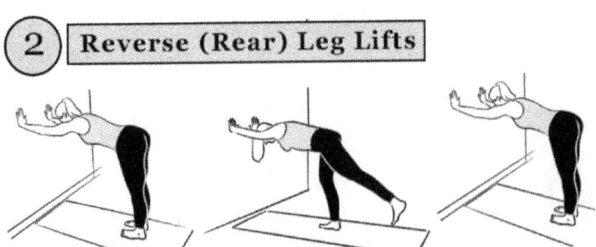

Start by facing the wall a bit more than an arm's length away. Bend at the waist keeping your body straight and put your palms on the wall bending until your body forms an "L". Keeping your hips pointing towards the floor, swing your right leg out behind you and up as far as you comfortably can. Hold for 1 second and bring back to the start position. That's one. Repeat for a total of ten repetitions then switch to the left leg for ten reps.

3. Wall Sit

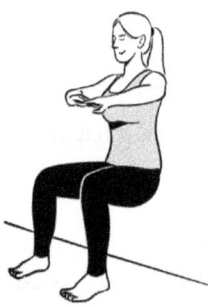

Stand with your back against the wall with your feet shoulder-width apart. walk your feet out slightly so that your back is leaning against the wall slightly. Slowly lower your body down the wall, keeping your feet flat on the floor. Stop when your thighs are parallel to the floor. If you can't see your toes, your feet are too far in towards the wall.. Stay in this parallel squat position for 30 seconds.

4. Wall-Supported Lunge

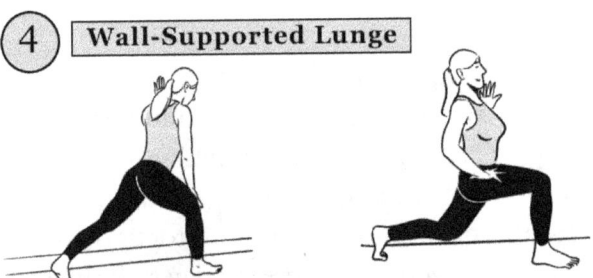

Stand next to the wall an arm's length away looking down the wall. Place your right hand on the wall and your left hand on your hips. Keeping you hips square, bend your left knee as you slide your right leg back behind you into a lunge position, bringing the knee down close to the floor. Hold momentarily, then press the left foot as you pull the right foot back in and squeeze your glutes back to the original position.

5. Wall-Facing Lunge

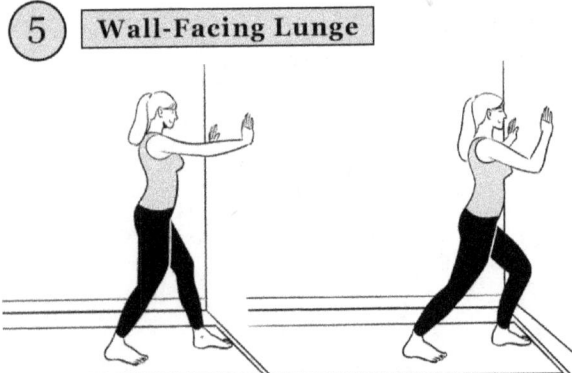

Face the wall and put your hands on it. Step your left foot forward, touching your toes to the wall, while your right foot goes backward. Bend both knees as you bring your left knee close to the wall. Avoid going too low, and keep your shoulders relaxed and your back and shoulders straight. Do five to ten reps, rest then repeat.

6. Child's Pose

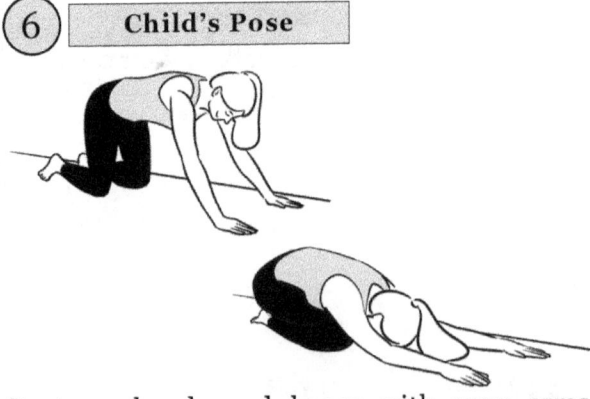

Start on hands and knees with your arms stretched out slightly in front of you. Bend back, bending your knees and folding your upper body so that you are almost sitting on your legs. Stretch out your arms in front of you with your head facing down and your palms on the floor. Hold for 20 seconds. Unwind, relax briefly and repeat one or two additional times.

LOWER-BODY EXERCISES 143

⑦ The Frog

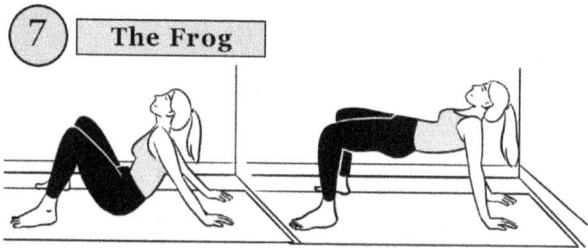

This is an advanced exercise, so start slow and stretch as much as you can without straining. The more you do the move, the farther you'll be able to stretch. Start in a tabletop or "crab walk" position: Your head, stomach and pelvis pointed towards the ceiling with your feet flat on the floor, knees bent and your hands behind you with your palms on the floor. Keep your arms fully extended and not bent. From here, push your buttocks up to straighten your back and stretch your spine as much as possible. Do this three to five times.

⑧ Floor Glute Bridge

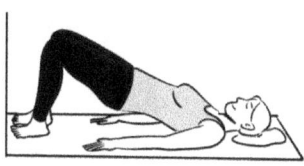

Lie on your back with your feet flat on the floor, toes touching the wall, and your knees bent at a 90-degree angle. Make sure your back is flat against the mat. Inhale slowly as you lift your hips towards the ceiling and squeeze your glutes. Hold for five seconds as you breathe out slowly, and breathe in slowly, return to start and relax briefly. Repeat ten times.

⑨ Mat Wall Bridge

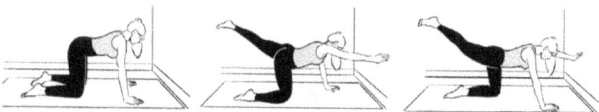

Start facing the wall, about an arm's length away, on your hands and knees. Simultaneously extend your left arm out to touch the wall and your right leg out behind you. Return and repeat with the other side: extend your right arm out to touch the wall and your left leg out behind you. Extend as far as you comfortably can without arching your back. Inhale as you extend the arm and leg, and exhale as you return to the starting position. Do 10-15 repetitions for each side, pause for 15 seconds and then repeat again.

⑩ Elevated Glute Bridge

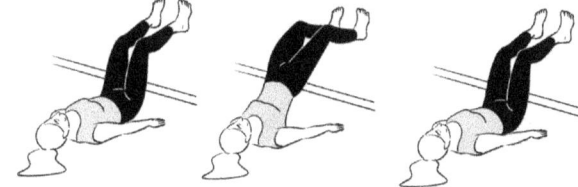

Lie faceup and place your feet flat on a wall about hip-width apart with your knees and hips bent at 90-degree angles and your arms extended along your sides. Action: Lift your hips until your body makes a straight line from your knees to your shoulders. Squeeze your glutes, then lower back to the floor.

⑪ Glute Bridge Cross

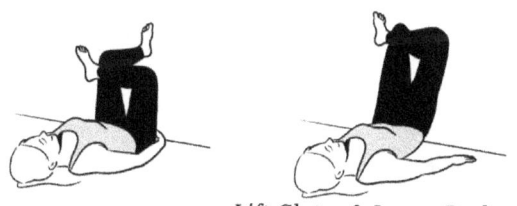

Lift Glutes & Lower Back

Lie on your back with your buttocks about a foot or so from the wall, your feet flat on the wall so that your lower legs are straight and your knees are bent at a 90-degree angle. Make sure your back is flat against the mat. Cross your right leg over your left, putting your right ankle on your left knee. Raise buttocks in a glute bridge position and hold for two seconds, then lower to mat. Repeat five times for each side.

⑫ Marching Glute Bridge

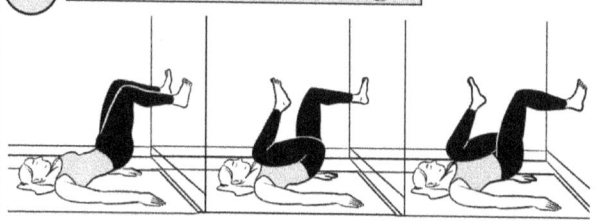

Lie on your back with your buttocks about a foot or so from the wall, your feet flat on the wall so that your lower legs are straight and your knees are bent at a 90-degree angle. Make sure your back is flat against the mat and your arms are along your sides. Lift your hips off the floor and bend your right knee towards your head while keeping your left foot on the wall. Put your right foot back on the wall and bend your left knee, lifting your left foot towards your head. That's one. Repeat 5-10 times.

13. Glute Bridge/Leg Raise

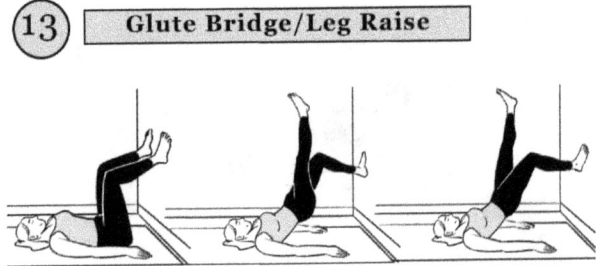

Lie on your back with your feet against the wall. Bend your knees to 90 degrees and extend your arms along your sides. Lift your glutes off the floor, and inhale as you raise your right leg up straight in the air. Your leg should be fully extended, and as close to your head as possible. Keep your head and shoulders firmly on the mat. Exhale as you return to the starting position and repeat with your left leg.

14. Split Stance Deadlift

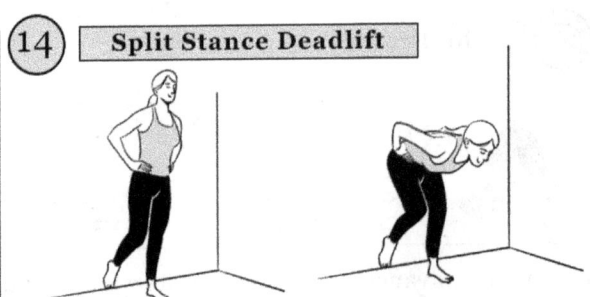

Stand with your back to the wall, both feet about a foot away. Place your right heel behind you on the wall with toes on the floor. With both knees slightly bent, bend at your hips keeping your back flat. Keep your front knee over your front ankle and tighten your core. Once your upper body is about parallel to floor, use your right foot to stand up, extending your hips. Do 8-10 reps. Then switch sides.

15. Side Step Against the Wall

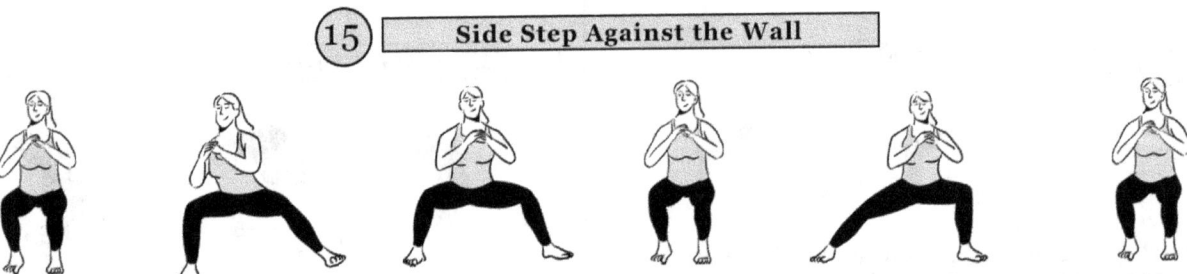

This is an advanced movement, so take it slow until you are used to the exercise. With this exercise, you are basically walking sideways against a wall in a squatted position. Start in a "wall sit" position with your back against the wall and your knees bent. Bend your elbows and clasp your hands in front of you. Slide your left foot and leg away from your right foot while keeping your body in the same position. Immediately bring your right foot and the rest of your body to the left back towards the other foot and leg so that you are again in a wall squat-your original position. Do this quickly for five steps to the left and then five steps back to the right. Rest momentarily and then repeat in both directions once more.

16. Calf Stretch

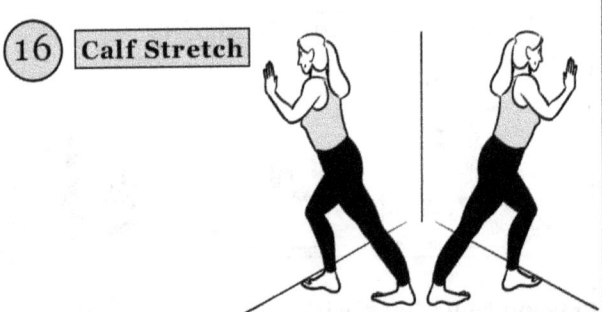

Stand facing the wall about 1-1/2 arms lengths away, feet shoulder length apart. Lean forward to the wall, bend your left knee as you slide the right foot back, keeping your foot flat on the floor until you feel the stretch in your calf. Hold for 10 seconds and release. Return to neutral position and repeat with the opposite leg and calf. An alternate method is to use a stair to stretch, hang your foot half way off of a stair and allow the heel to drop below the stair to stretch.

17. Calf Raises/Bent Leg

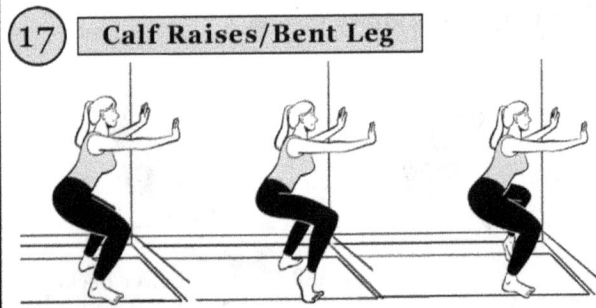

Stand facing the wall, an arm's length away with your palms on the wall and feet wide apart. Turn your toes outward and bend your knees to lower down to a 90-degree angle at the knees. Alternate raising heels off the floor: right-left-right-left. Do 15-20 right-left reps then return to starting position. For a more challenging exercise, stretch at the top by holding your heel off the floor for five seconds before returning it to the floor.

18. Mountain Climber

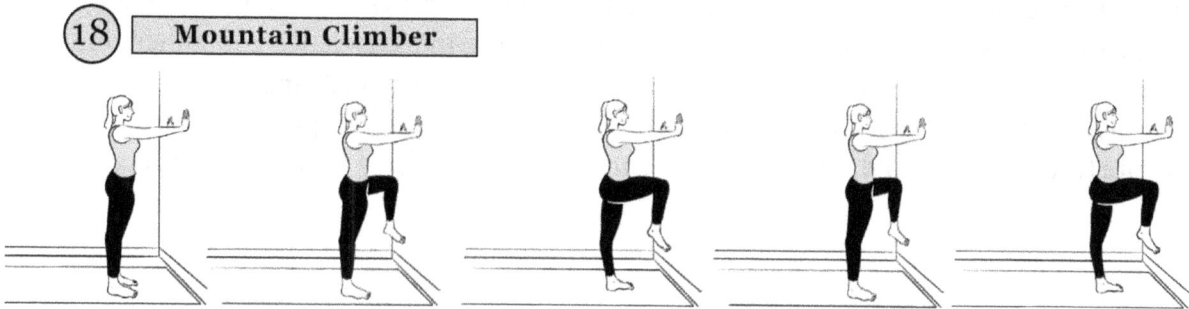

Stand an arm's length away with your hands on the wall and your arms fully extended but not bent. To start, bend your leg and lift your right knee towards the wall with your toes and lower leg pointed down. Immediately return to start and repeat with the left leg, while keeping your back straight. The movements should be controlled, but quick. Repeat the back-and-forth motion for 10-15 repetitions. For a more difficult exercise, move back two steps so that you are leaning towards the wall and follow the same instructions above, being careful not to bend your back while stepping.

19. Windshield Wipers

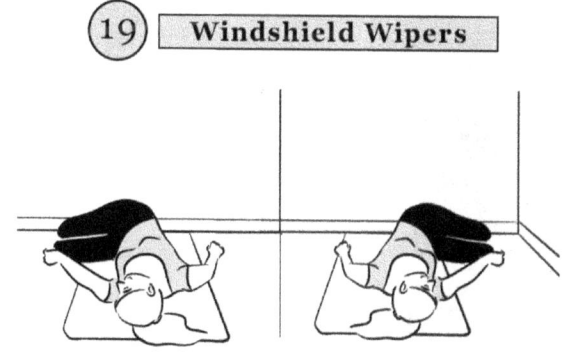

Start on your back with your arms to your side, knees bent and your feet flat on the wall for spacing. Bring your knees toward your chest slightly and roll your legs to the left until they touch the floor. Hold momentarily and then roll them back to the right until they touch the floor on the right. That's one. Repeat five to ten times. For a more difficult exercise, perform with legs almost straight.

20. Hip Flexors with Chair

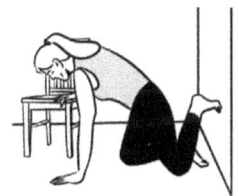 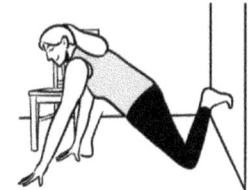 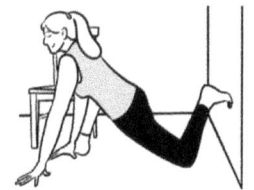 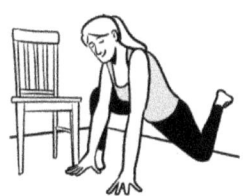

With a chair sideways in front of you, kneel down with your back to and your feet touching the wall. Lean forward so your right hand is on the chair seat for support and your left hand is on the floor. Place your left foot on the wall with the ball of your foot touching. Bring your right foot forward and bend your knee so that your foot is flat on the floor. Next, put your right hand on the floor and gently push your pelvis forward and away from the wall to feel the stretch. Hold for 3-5 seconds and then slightly twist your hips and pelvis to the right as you lift your head. Hold until you feel the muscles loosen (about 10 seconds). Unwind and repeat with the opposite leg on the wall.

That's it for exercises focusing on the lower body. The exercises we've explored here are more than just routines; they're powerful tools for maintaining independence and enhancing your quality of life. Use them to target your lower body and for personalizing the 28-Day Success Plan to your specific needs. And remember, your goal shouldn't be perfection, but rather to cultivate functional strength that supports your lifestyle and helps you stay active and able to do the activities you love.

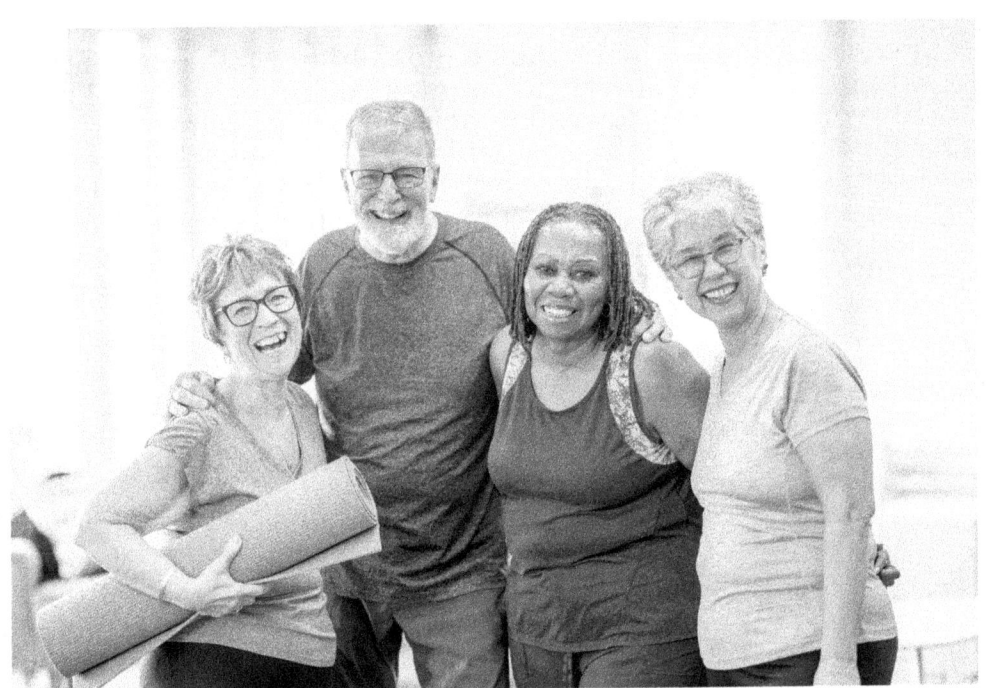

CHAPTER 12
Exercises for Mobility and Independence

• • • ● • ● • • •

In this chapter we're focusing on Hip Flexors and Glutes. The Hip Flexors are a group of muscles located at the front of your hip that allow you to lift your knee towards your chest and bend at the waist. They together with the Glutes, which are the large muscles in your buttocks. While the Hip Flexors are responsible for lifting your legs, the Glutes help extend the hips and rotate the thighs. They come into play for standing up, walking and bending; so they're pretty important! When they're strong and flexible, they provide stability to your pelvis and lower back, reducing the risk of pain, injury, and falls.

By focusing on exercises that strengthen and stretch both the Hip Flexors and Glutes in this chapter, we're aiming to significantly enhance our mobility, reduce our fall risk, and maintain an active, independent lifestyle as long as possible.

As with the previous chapters, this one is also for "do it yourself" exercising where you can customize your own routines. Pick five or six exercises from this group to do as one routine for targeting mobility and independence. Rotate exercises in and out from the group each time you do a targeted routine. Some exercises cross over from other chapters due to their benefits to multiple parts of the body. Remember to always talk to your doctor before starting any exercise program, including this one.

We'll get started with warm-ups then move right into the main routines.

Exercises for Mobility & Independence

1. Arm Raises Against Wall

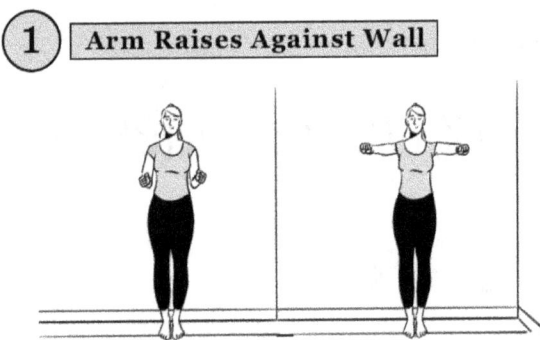

Stand upright with your back against the wall so that your head, buttocks, and upper back are firmly pressed against it. Your feet should not be too far apart. Bend your elbows to form a 90° angle. Raise your arms and begin the movement, sliding your elbows along your sides. Keep your arms and back against the wall at all times. Inhale when raising your arms and exhale when returning to the starting position.

2. Wall Sit

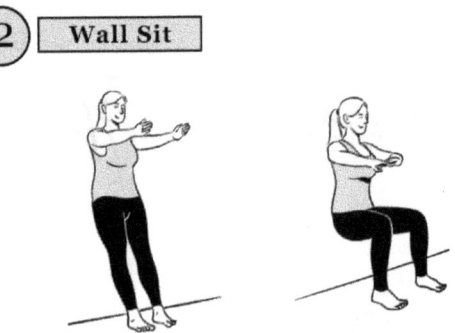

Stand with your back against the wall with your feet shoulder-width apart. walk your feet out slightly so that your back is leaning against the wall slightly. Slowly lower your body down the wall, keeping your feet flat on the floor. Stop when your thighs are parallel to the floor. If you can't see your toes, your feet are too far in towards the wall. Stay in this parallel squat position for 30 seconds.

3. Hip Circles

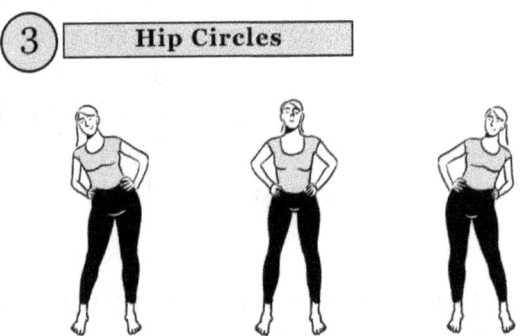

Stand facing the wall, with your feet spread shoulder-width apart and about two feet away from the wall. Put your hands on your hips and pull your stomach in so that you engage your core muscle. Bend to the side slightly as you rotate your hips clockwise 10 times at a medium speed. Repeat in the opposite direction.

4. Side Bend/Side Stretch

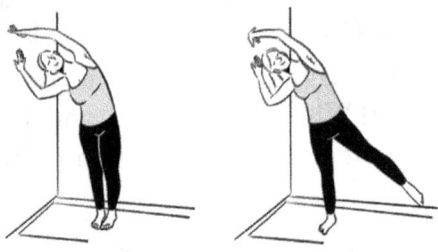

Begin by standing sideways arm's length from the wall, with your right side closest to the wall and feet hip-width apart. Put your right forearm on the wall, extend your left arm overhead, and slide your right hand down the wall as you bend your torso to the right. Hold this position while lifting your left leg up and out sideways for ten repetitions. Switch sides and repeat.

5. Fwd Bend/Side Leg Lift

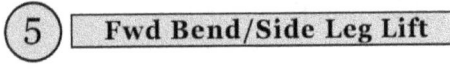
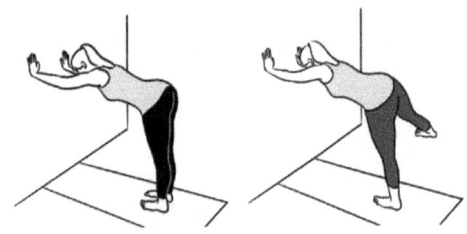

Stand facing the wall and bend forward until your torso is parallel to the floor, your arms straight, and your palms flat against the wall. Lift your left leg out to the side until it's parallel to the floor (or as high as you can), keeping your hips level. Do 10 repetitions and repeat with the right leg.

6. Wall-Facing Lunge

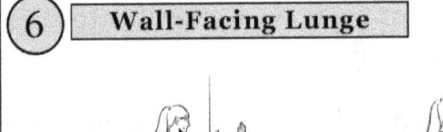
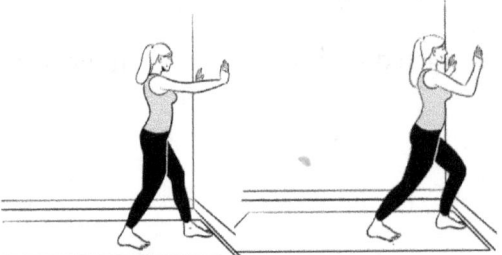

Start by facing the wall a little more than an arm's length away. Lean over and place your hands on the wall without bending your knees. Keeping your feet in place, slowly bend at the knees towards the wall and hold momentarily before coming back to the starting position. Do this 5-10 times.

EXERCISES FOR MOBILITY AND INDEPENDENCE 149

7. Press lunge

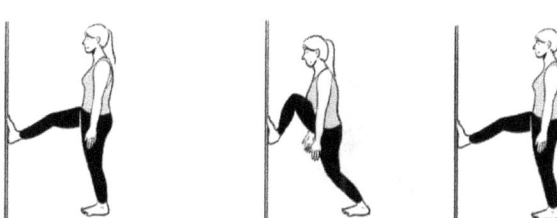

Begin by standing one leg-length away from a wall. Balance yourself, then place one foot on the wall at hip-height. Bend your knee and lunge forward until your quad is in line with your core, keeping your torso neutral and upright. Pause for 1 Second, then press through the ball of your foot to return to your starting position. Repeat for each set.

8. Standing Side Lunge

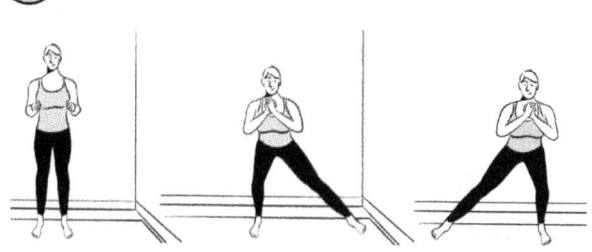

With your back to the wall, clasp your hands in front of you with your elbows bent. Slide your left foot to the left and bend your left knee while keeping your right leg straight and in place on the floor. Hold momentarily and return to center. Repeat on the opposite side.

9. Knee Raise on Mat

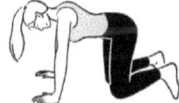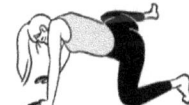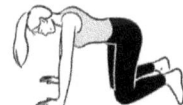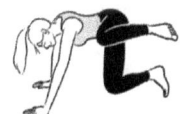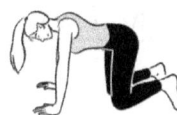

Get on your hands and knees with your feet slightly touching the wall behind you. Keeping your back and arms straight and knee bent, lift your right leg out first towards the right then up towards the ceiling. Hold momentarily and then back to the floor. Repeat five to ten times on each side by either alternating legs or doing five to ten reps on each side before switching.

10. Multi-Stretch

Start on your knees parallel to the wall. Stretch your left leg out in front of you with your leg bent and the foot flat on the floor. Lean forward with your torso to add a stretch to the planted knee's hip flexor. Place one hand on the floor opposite to the front foot. Finally, reach your left arm up and rotate towards the ceiling leading with your upper back and shoulders. Hold for 3 seconds then repeat on the opposite side.

11. Forward Squat

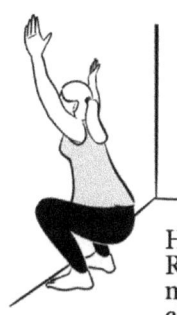

Start facing the wall with your feet shoulder length apart and your toes about a foot from the wall. Keeping you head up, lift your arms above your head and squat down until your thighs are parallel with the floor. Hold for a second, push back up. Repeat 8-10 times. As you get more comfortable, put your feet closer to the wall, but make sure to keep your back straight and your head up.

12. Single Leg Squat

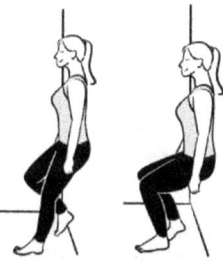

Start with your back on the wall and your feet about one foot from it with your arms at your side. Bend your right leg to lift your foot off the ground slightly so that your weight is on your left foot. Bend your left knee as you squat down, keeping your left foot flat on the floor and your right foot elevated. Stop and hold before your leg is parallel to the floor. Push back up and repeat five times. Switch and repeat with the right leg bearing your weight.

13. Squat with Cactus Arms

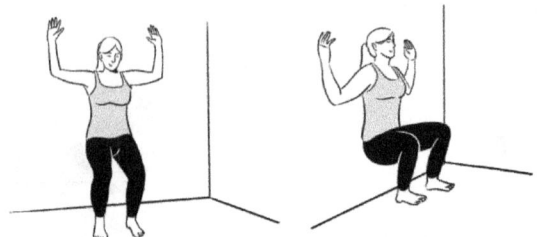

Stand with your back against the wall and bend your elbows so your hands are pointing up like a cartoon cactus. Walk your feet out in front slightly then slide down into a squat by bending your knees until your thighs are parallel with the floor while keeping your elbows against the wall. Hold momentarily and then push back to your original position. Repeat for 5-10 repetitions.

14. Balance Bear

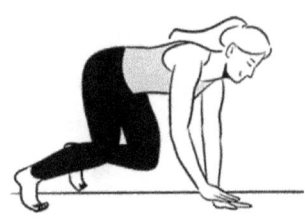

Start on your hands and feet like a bear. Keep your back straight. From this position, lift your right hand and your left foot off the floor an inch or two, then replace. Repeat with other side: lift your left hand and your right foot off the floor an inch or two then replace. That's one repetition. Do a total of five to ten repetitions.

15. Bear Walk-Forwards

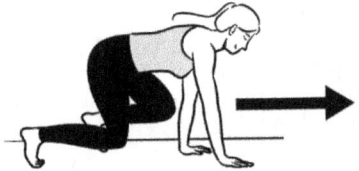

This is the "Balance Bear", but instead of staying in one spot, you actually "walk" forward across the floor. Start on your hands and feet like a bear. Keep your back straight and slowly walk across the floor in the balance bear stance. Pause, then retrace your steps backwards to your starting spot. Do a total of four repetitions.

16. Bear Walk-Backwards

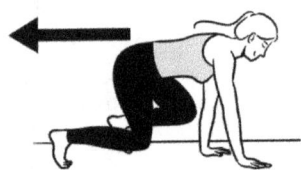

This is the "Balance Walk" in reverse. It is meant to be performed together with the Forward Bear Walk. After walking forward on your hands and feet, walk backwards to your starting spot. Keep your back straight and slowly walk across the floor in the balance bear stance. Pause, then retrace your steps forward. Do a total of four reps.

17. Bear Walk-Sideways

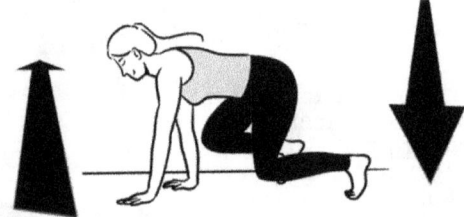

This is the "Bear Walk" to the sides. Start on your hands and feet like a bear. Keep your back straight and slowly walk sideways in the bear walk stance going first left to right then retracing your steps right to left to your starting position. Do a grand total of four repetitions.

18. Bear Walk-Circle

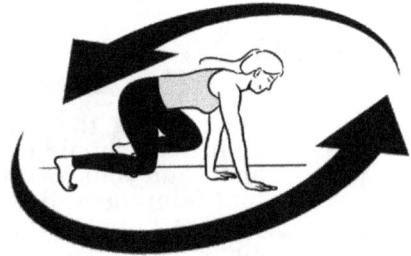

This is the "Bear Walk" in a circle. Start on your hands and feet like a bear. Keep your back straight and slowly walk clockwise in a circle in the bear walk stance. Do four rotations in each direction. To avoid getting dizzy, move slowly and rest in-between if necessary.

19) Split Squat

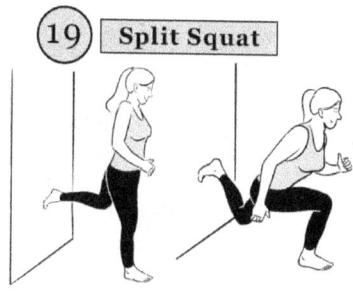

Stand facing away from the wall about three feet away. Bend your knee and place your left foot on the wall behind you. Using your arms to balance, bend down into a squatting position while keeping your left leg foot on the wall. Immediately return to the starting position. Quickly do 8-10 reps and then switch legs.

20) Reverse Lunge

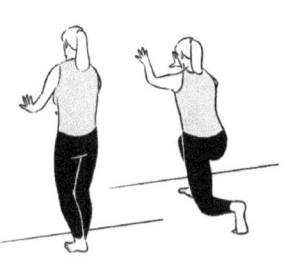

Stand facing the wall, an arm's length away, and your feet a few inches apart. Place your hands against the wall, bend your right knee as you step backwards with your left leg into a lunge. Go as far back as possible with your right knee never going beyond the toes. Return to the starting position, and repeat on the opposite side. Avoid arching your back, and don't lean too far forward. Do this five times on each side.

21) Hip Flexor with Chair

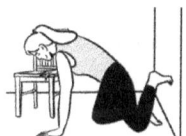 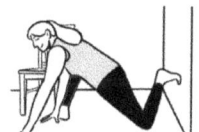 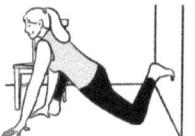 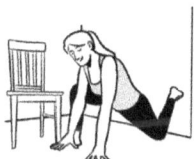

With a chair sideways in front of you, kneel down with your back to and your feet touching the wall. Lean forward so your right hand is on the chair seat for support and your left hand is on the floor. Place your left foot on the wall with the ball of your foot touching. Bring your right foot forward and bend your knee so that your foot is flat on the floor. Next, put your right hand on the floor and gently push your pelvis forward and away from the wall to feel the stretch. Hold for 3-5 seconds and then slightly twist your hips and pelvis to the right as you lift your head. Hold until you feel the muscles loosen (about 10 seconds). Unwind and repeat with the opposite leg on the wall.

22) Side Step

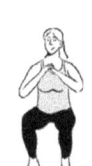 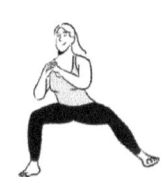 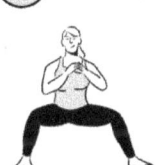 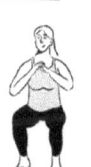 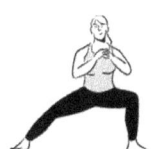 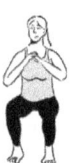

Start in a "Wall Sit" position with your back against the wall and your knees bent. Bend your elbows and clasp your hands in front of you. Slide your left foot and leg away from your right foot while keeping your body in the same position. Immediately bring your right foot and the rest of your body to the left back towards the other foot and leg so that you are again in a wall squat-your original position. Do this quickly for five steps to the left and then five steps back to the right. Rest momentarily and then repeat in both directions once more.

23) Lunge Twist

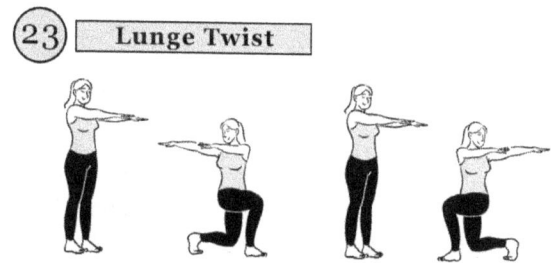

Stand three feet from the wall facing away with your arms extended in front. Bend your left leg backward so that your foot touches the wall. Then, lunge and squat forward with your right leg while twisting your torso to the right. Hold briefly and return to a standing position. Repeat five times then change to the left side.

24) Wall Scissors

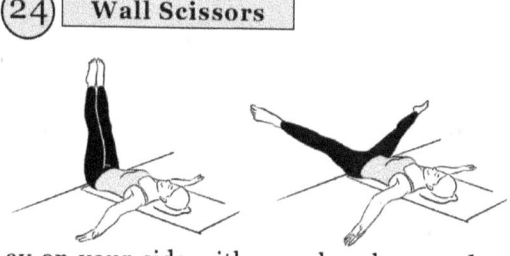

Lay on your side with your legs bent and against the wall. Roll over onto your back so that your legs and buttocks are up against the wall. Stretch your arms out from your side like an airplane. Open your legs widely to stretch the inner thigh and hold for two seconds. Bring back to neutral. Repeat 10 times.

(18) Mountain Climber

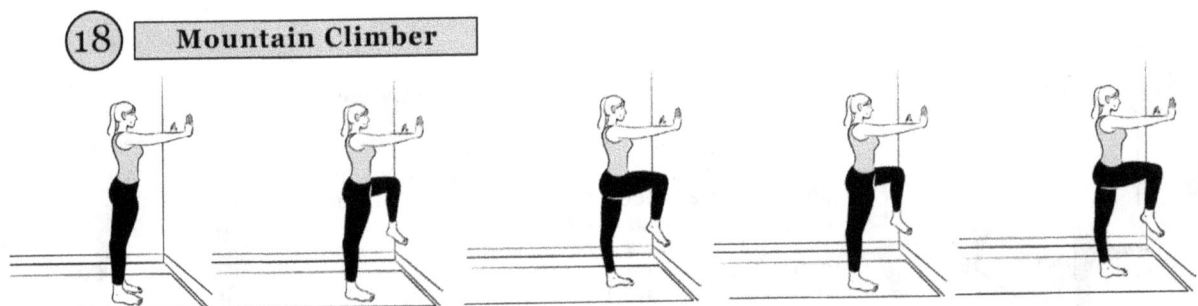

Stand an arm's length away with your hands on the wall and your arms fully extended but not bent. To start, bend your leg and lift your right knee towards the wall with your toes and lower leg pointed down. Immediately return to start and repeat with the left leg, while keeping your back straight. The movements should be controlled, but quick. Repeat the back-and-forth motion for 10-15 repetitions. For a more difficult exercise, move back two steps so that you are leaning towards the wall and follow the same instructions above, being careful not to bend your back while stepping.

(19) Windshield Wipers

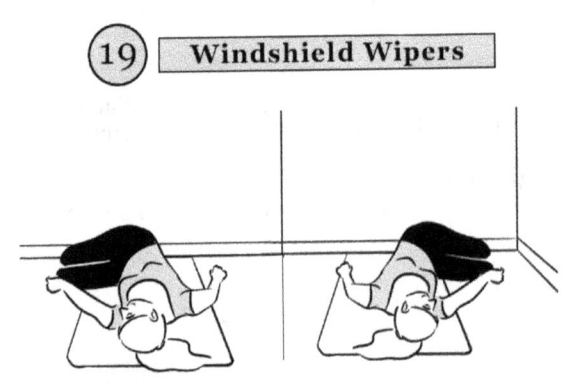

Start on your back with your arms to your side, knees bent and your feet flat on the wall for spacing. Bring your knees toward your chest slightly and roll your legs to the left until they touch the floor. Hold momentarily and then roll them back to the right until they touch the floor on the right. That's one. Repeat five to ten times. For a more difficult exercise, perform with legs almost straight.

(20) Hip Flexors with Chair

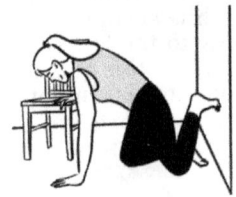 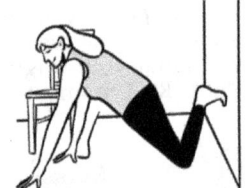 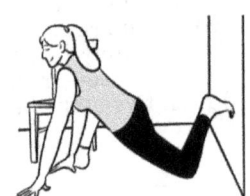 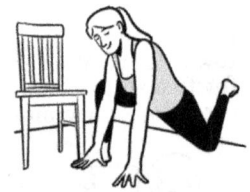

With a chair sideways in front of you, kneel down with your back to and your feet touching the wall. Lean forward so your right hand is on the chair seat for support and your left hand is on the floor. Place your left foot on the wall with the ball of your foot touching. Bring your right foot forward and bend your knee so that your foot is flat on the floor. Next, put your right hand on the floor and gently push your pelvis forward and away from the wall to feel the stretch. Hold for 3-5 seconds and then slightly twist your hips and pelvis to the right as you lift your head. Hold until you feel the muscles loosen (about 10 seconds). Unwind and repeat with the opposite leg on the wall.

That's it for Chapter 12 and our exercises for mobility and independence. It's never too late to start, and even small, consistent efforts can lead to remarkable improvements in your strength, flexibility, and balance. For a more comprehensive and overarching workout, continue using the "28-Day Success Plan" in Chapters 6 and 7 for overall body fitness and strength.

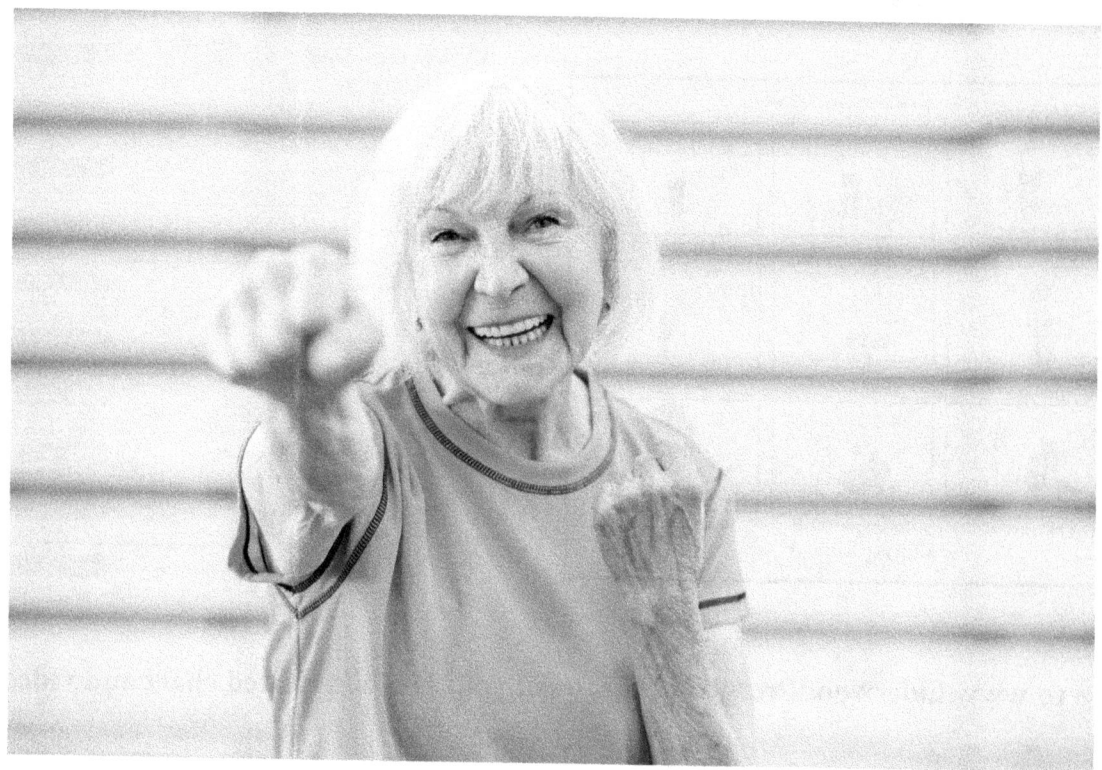

Free Illustration Chart

Free Video Demonstrations

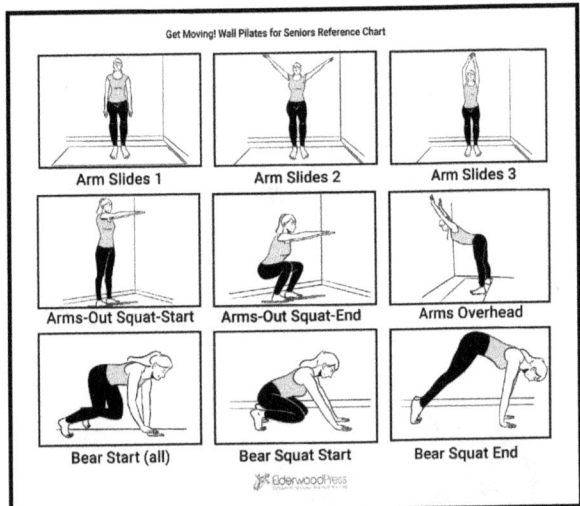

Master Video	WATCH VIDEO >
Warm-Ups	WATCH VIDEO >
Success Plan Part 1	WATCH VIDEO >
Success Plan Part 2	WATCH VIDEO >
Strength & Fitness	WATCH VIDEO >
Upper Body Exercises	WATCH VIDEO >
Lower Body Exercises	WATCH VIDEO >
Core Exercises (Bonus Video)	WATCH VIDEO >
Balance & Coordination	WATCH VIDEO >
Exercises for Independence (Bonus Video)	WATCH VIDEO >

Go to www.ElderwoodPress.com/wp to get your free illustrated chart and videos.

CHAPTER 13
Our Gifts to You

• • • ● • ● • ● • ● • ● •

Starting any exercise routine can be daunting. That's why we've put together a series of FREE VIDEOS that show you how to do each exercise properly.

Free Illustration Chart

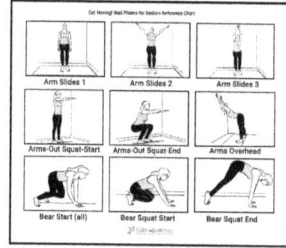

Free Video Demonstrations

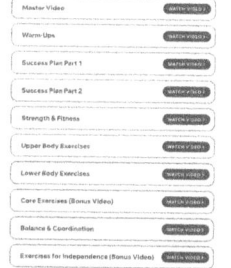

In addition, you can download our free reference chart with illustrations of the exercises used in this book. Just go to: www.elderwoodpress.com/wp, enter your email there and we'll send you access to the reference chart and videos.

Now that you've made it through your first month, we hope you will continue on your journey of continued strength and fitness. And remember, if you feel your motivation waning, here are a few things you can do to jumpstart your workouts again.

Recognize the Signs of a Plateau

When your progress seems to stall or "plateau", it usually means that your body has adapted to the current routine. This can be frustrating and make you want to quit. To counteract this, do something different. For instance, you can change the order of your routines or add weights or resistance bands to make the exercises more difficult. Try changing your hand or foot placement to subtly increase the difficulty, or substitute exercises from the targeted routines (chapters 8-12) to personalize your 28-Day Success Plan. As long as it doesn't adversely affect the exercises, it may get you past the plateau and on to the next hill.

Set Realistic Goals

Establish short-term goals that you can realistically reach to keep your motivation high and help you feel a sense of accomplishment. For instance, improved alignment, increased reps, or adding exercises to an existing routine. Long-term goals should align with your personal values and lifestyle aspirations, like "maintaining independence" or "enhancing the quality of your life".

Overcome Mental Barriers

Mental fatigue or lack of confidence can often be just as limiting as physical barriers when it comes to exercise. Being "mindful" or "in the moment" and using positive self-talk can combat negative thoughts that might hinder your motivation. Boredom with the routine can lead to a lack of enthusiasm. Once you are comfortable, add or remove exercises to mix things up. Make other low-impact activities such as swimming or walking part of your overall routine to help keep you engaged. This is why we encourage alternate forms of exercise on your "rest days".

Movement is essential for a healthy and fulfilling life, no matter how old you are. The exercises we've presented here are aimed at helping you maintain and enhance your fitness, strength, balance, and overall well-being. By weaving these activities into your daily routine, you're investing in your health and enriching your quality of life. And remember: every small step matters! Even if you can't quite master all the exercises right away, the key is to stay active and progress at a pace that feels right for you. Listen to your body, celebrate the little victories and consistently push on. And keep in mind that physical activity benefits not just your body but also your mind. Staying active stimulates your brain, boosts your mood, and can help you maintain your independence.

You've started on a "holistic journey" that connects mind, body, and lifestyle. Now start incorporating core engagement and posture awareness into your daily activities—sit upright while driving or clinch and tighten your core muscles while standing in line. Pick a few breathing exercises and add them to your morning wake-up ritual. Try setting a specific time each day for practice.

Get moving and keep moving-it's just the beginning of your new fitness journey!

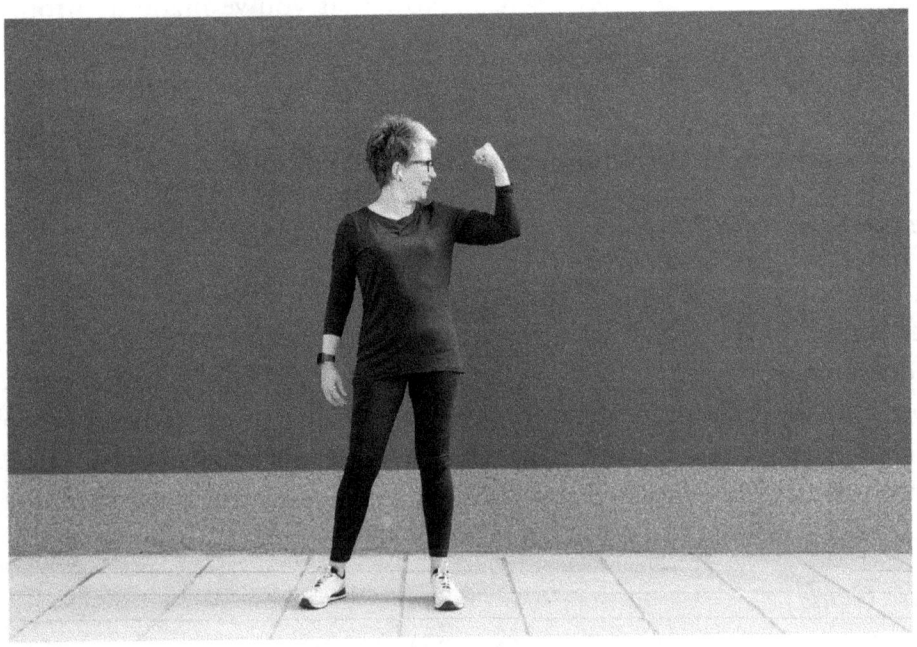

We would love to hear from you!

It's through your support and reviews that my book is able to reach others who can benefit from its content. Please take 60 seconds to kindly leave a review on Amazon by scanning the QR code below. If you live in a country that isn't listed, please use the link provided in your Amazon order.

Please follow these steps to rate/review this book:

1. Open the camera on your phone
2. Hover it over the QR code
3. Rate/review my book on Amazon
4. Or go to https://amzn.to/4id1UJv

Thank you!

Other Books from Elderwood Press

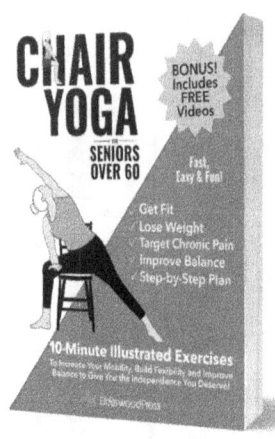

Chair Yoga
for Seniors Over 60
(With FREE Videos!)

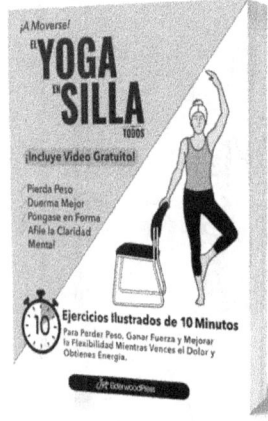

El Yoga en Silla
Para Todos

(¡Incluye Video Gratis!)

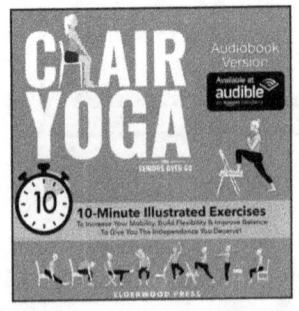

Chair Yoga
for Seniors Over 60
(Audiobook)

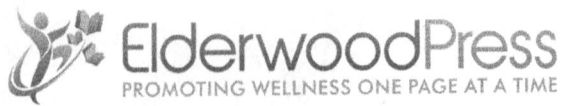

Glossary

A list of terms used in this book.

Abs (Abdominals): Located on the front of the torso, they stabilize the core and assist in bending and rotating the trunk.

Abductors: Muscles on the outer thigh that move the leg away from the middle of the body. Important for sideways leg movements and balance.

Adductors: Inner thigh muscles that pull the legs towards the middle of the body. Used for walking and stabilizing the pelvis.

Biceps: Located on the front of the upper arm, they flex the elbow and rotate the forearm. Used in lifting and pulling actions.

Calves: Muscles at the back of the lower leg, responsible for pointing the toes, walking and running.

Cardio: Related to the heart. In this book, cardio refers to exercise that gets the heart pumping above a normal resting rate.

Core: The muscles of the abdomen, lower back, and pelvis that stabilize the spine and pelvis during movement.

Deltoids: Shoulder muscles responsible for arm raising and rotation.

Fitness: How well your body can handle everyday activities and challenges, like walking, running, playing sports, or just keeping up with your friends without getting overly tired.

Glutes: Buttocks muscles, crucial for hip extension, climbing stairs, and maintaining posture.

Groin: Area between the abdomen and thigh, contains muscles involved in leg adduction and hip flexion. Important for stability and mobility.

Hamstrings: Muscles at the back of the thigh. These flex the knee and extend the hip, important for walking, running and climbing.

Hip Flexor: Muscles that bring the thigh towards the torso. Used for walking, climbing and running.

Inner Thigh: aka Adductors. Muscles that pull the legs towards the middle of the body. Used for walking and stabilizing the pelvis.

Lats (Latissimus Dorsi): Large back muscles that pull the arms down and back, involved in many pulling movements.

Love Handles: Slang for fat deposits on the sides of the waist.

Mobility: How easily and safely you can move around to do the normal things you need to do every day.

Obliques: Side abdominal muscles that rotate and bend the trunk. Important for bending.

Pectorals, or Pecs: Large muscles of the chest, involved in pushing movements and arm adduction.

Pelvis: Bony structure that connects the spine to the legs, crucial for weight transfer, stability and mobility.

Quadriceps: Four muscles on the front of the thigh that extend the knee, essential for walking, running, and jumping.

Reps & Sets: A rep is one complete motion of an exercise. A set is a group of consecutive reps performed without resting. Reps are counted individually within a set, while sets count groups of reps. You typically rest between sets, not between individual reps.

Scapula: Shoulder blade, a flat bone on the back of the shoulder that serves as an attachment point for many muscles.

Strength: The amount of power your muscles have to lift, push, or move things.

Thoracic Spine: Middle segment of the spine, involved in trunk rotation and rib cage movements.

Trapezius or "Traps": Large upper back and neck muscle, involved in shoulder blade movement and head positioning.

Triceps: Muscle on the back of the upper arm that extends the elbow, used in pushing movements.

References

References appear in alphabetical order.

12 Scientifically Proven Benefits of Pilates for Your Peace of Mind. (2013, September 25). Pilates Bridge. https://pilatesbridge.com/12-scientifically-proven-benefits-of-pilates-for-your-peace-of-mind/

A Step-by-Step guide on promoting heart health for seniors. (n.d.). https://www.springhills.com/resources/heart-health-for-seniors

Admin. (2020, July 29). *What is metabolism? - definition, types, process.* BYJUS. https://byjus.com/biology/metabolism/

Caldwell, K., Adams, M., Quin, R., Harrison, M., & Greeson, J. (2013). Pilates, Mindfulness and Somatic Education. *Journal of Dance & Somatic Practices,* 5(2), 141–153. https://www.ncbi.nlm.nih.gov/pmc/articles/PMC4198945/

Cannataro, R., Cione, E., Bonilla, D. A., Cerullo, G., Angelini, F., & D'Antona, G. (2022). Strength training in elderly: A useful tool against sarcopenia. *Frontiers in Sports and Active Living,* 4(950949), 950949. https://doi.org/10.3389/fspor.2022.950949

Centers for Disease Control and Prevention. (2020, November 23). *Older Adult Falls Data.* Www.cdc.gov. https://www.cdc.gov/falls/data/index.html

Department of Health & Human Services. (n.d.). *Metabolism.* Better Health Channel. https://www.betterhealth.vic.gov.au/health/conditionsandtreatments/metabolism

For older adults, every 500 additional steps taken daily associated with lower heart risk. (n.d.). American Heart Association. https://newsroom.heart.org/news/for-older-adults-every-500-additional-steps-taken-daily-associated-with-lower-heart-risk

Good Pain vs. Bad Pain » Arthritis, Exercise, & Active Living: The ENACT Center | Boston University. (n.d.). Www.bu.edu. https://www.bu.edu/enact/living-well/exercise-and-arthritis/exercises/good-pain-vs-bad-pain/

Harbour, E., Stöggl, T., Schwameder, H., & Finkenzeller, T. (2022). Breath Tools: A synthesis of Evidence-Based breathing Strategies to enhance human running. Frontiers in Physiology, 13. https://doi.org/10.3389/fphys.2022.813243

Harvard Health. (2016, February 19). *Preserve your muscle mass* https://www.health.harvard.edu/staying-healthy/preserve-your-muscle-mass

Illidi, C. R., Romer, L. M., Johnson, M. A., Williams, N. C., Rossiter, H. B., Casaburi, R., & Tiller, N. B. (2023). Distinguishing science from pseudoscience in commercial respiratory interventions: an evidence-based guide for health and exercise professionals. *European Journal of Applied Physiology, 123*(8), 1599–1625. https://doi.org/10.1007/s00421-023-05166-8

Ioannou, E., Chen, H. L., Bromley, V., Fosker, S., Ali, K., Fernando, A., Mensah, E., & Fowler-Davis, S. (2023). The key values and factors identified by older adults to promote physical activity and reduce sedentary behaviour using co-production approaches: a scoping review. *BMC Geriatrics, 23*(1). https://doi.org/10.1186/s12877-023-04005-x

Kloubec, J. (2011). Pilates: how does it work and who needs it? *Muscles, Ligaments and Tendons Journal, 1*(2), 61–66. https://www.ncbi.nlm.nih.gov/pmc/articles/PMC3666467/

Lichtenstein, A. H., Appel, L. J., Vadiveloo, M., Hu, F. B., Kris-Etherton, P. M., Rebholz, C. M., Sacks, F. M., Thorndike, A. N., Van Horn, L., & Wylie-Rosett, J. (2021). 2021 Dietary Guidance to Improve Cardiovascular Health: A scientific statement from the American Heart Association. *Circulation, 144*(23). https://doi.org/10.1161/cir.0000000000001031

Lifestyle and Management options for Physical Activity | American Geriatrics Society | HealthInAging.org. (n.d.). Www.healthinaging.org. https://www.healthinaging.org/a-z-topic/physical-activity/lifestyle

Lim, E.-J., & Hyun, E.-J. (2021). The Impacts of Pilates and Yoga on Health-Promoting Behaviors and Subjective Health Status. *International Journal of Environmental Research and Public Health, 18*(7), 3802. https://doi.org/10.3390/ijerph18073802

Mazzeo, R. S., Cavanagh, P., Evans, W. J., Fiatarone, M., Hagberg, J., McAuley, E., & Startzell, J. (1998). ACSM Position Stand: Exercise and Physical Activity for Older Adults. *Medicine & Science in Sports & Exercise, 30*(6), 992–1008. https://journals.lww.com/acsm-msse/fulltext/1998/06000/acsm_position_stand__exercise_and_physical.33.aspx

metabolism. (n.d.). Britannica Kids. https://kids.britannica.com/kids/article/metabolism/603299

Metabolism: Medline Plus Medical Encyclopedia. (n.d.). https://medlineplus.gov/ency/article/002257.htm

Metabolism. (2024). In *Merriam-Webster Dictionary.* https://www.merriam-webster.com/dictionary/metabolism

Meredith, S. J., Cox, N. J., Ibrahim, K., Higson, J., McNiff, J., Mitchell, S., Rutherford, M., Wijayendran, A., Shenkin, S. D., Kilgour, A. H. M., & Lim, S. E. R. (2023). Factors that influence older adults' participation in physical activity: a systematic review of qualitative studies. *Age And Ageing, 52*(8).https://doi.org/10.1093/ageing/afad145

Mesinovic, J., Fyfe, J. J., Talevski, J., Wheeler, M. J.,Leung, G. K., George, E. S., Hunegnaw, M. T., Glavas, C., Jansons, P., Daly, R.M., & Scott, D. (2023). Type 2 Diabetes mellitus and sarcopenia as comorbidChronic diseases in Older adults: Established and Emerging Treatments andtherapies. *Diabetes & Metabolism Journal, 47*(6), 719–742.https://doi.org/10.4093/dmj.2023.0112

Modern Heart and Vascular. (2024, August 4). *Senior HeartHealth - modern heart and vascular*.https://www.modernheartandvascular.com/senior-heart-health/

Newell, T. (2024, January 3). *6 Reasons to Give Pilates a Try*. AARP; AARP.https://www.aarp.org/health/healthy-living/info-2024/pilates-wellness-benefits.html

Ogle, M. (2021, May 21). *The 6 essential principles of pilates.* Verywell Fit.https://www.verywellfit.com/six-pilates-principles-2704854

Pereira, M. J.,Mendes, R., Mendes, R. S., Martins, F., Gomes, R., Gama, J., Dias, G., &Castro, M. A. (2022). Benefits of Pilates in the Elderly Population: ASystematic Review and Meta-Analysis. *EuropeanJournal of Investigation in Health, Psychology and Education, 12*(3), 236–268.https://doi.org/10.3390/ejihpe12030018

Pilates and weightloss. (2023, May 9). Www.medicalnewstoday.com.https://www.medicalnewstoday.com/articles/is-pilates-good-for-weight-loss

Potočnik, M. M.,Edwards, I., & Potočnik, N. (2023). Locomotor–Respiratory Entrainment uponPhonated Compared to Spontaneous Breathing during Submaximal Exercise. International Journal of EnvironmentalResearch and Public Health, 20(4),2838. https://doi.org/10.3390/ijerph20042838

Strong, R. (2023, July 29). *10 fitness goals, recommended by personal trainers*. Health. https://www.health.com/fitness/fitness-goals

The impact of Pilateson the postural alignment of healthy adules. (2016, December). Revista Brasileira de Medicinado Esporte.https://www.researchgate.net/publication/312061661_The_impact_of_pilates_exercises_on_the_postural_alignment_of_healthy_adults

Wu, S., Li, G., Shi, B., Ge, H., Chen, S., Zhang, X., &He, Q. (2024). Comparative effectiveness of interventions on promoting physicalactivity in older adults: A systematic review and network meta-analysis. *DigitalHealth, 10*. https://doi.org/10.1177/20552076241239182

Zaccaro, A., Piarulli, A., Laurino, M., Garbella, E.,Menicucci, D., Neri, B., & Gemignani, A. (2018). How Breath-Control CanChange Your Life: A systematic review on Psycho-Physiological correlates of slow breathing. *Frontiers in Human Neuroscience, 12*.https://doi.org/10.3389/fnhum.2018.00353

www.ingramcontent.com/pod-product-compliance
Lightning Source LLC
Chambersburg PA
CBHW080518030426
42337CB00023B/4565